A Quiet Courage

A Quiet Courage

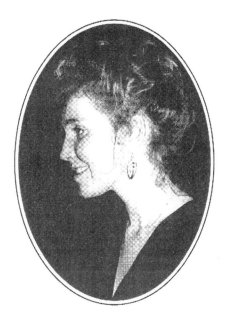

The moving story of a young girl's courageous battle against cancer, as told by her father

Jim McCallum

authorHOUSE®

AuthorHouse™
1663 Liberty Drive
Bloomington, IN 47403
www.authorhouse.com
Phone: 1-800-839-8640

Edited by Carol Bell.

First published by AuthorHouse   08/19/2011

ISBN: 978-1-4567-9366-1 (sc)
ISBN: 978-1-4567-9365-4 (ebk)

Printed in the United States of America

Any people depicted in stock imagery provided by Thinkstock are models, and such images are being used for illustrative purposes only.
Certain stock imagery © Thinkstock.

This book is printed on acid-free paper.

Contents

The world is our stage, we are the actors

Every one of us who have lost our children

We play so many parts in public

Nobody can tell what goes on under the painted smile.

In private the paint cracks, the tears fall

Another day dawns, put on your make up, and painted smile

No one sees beneath the facade

After a while, does anyone care?

Yes, I'm sure they do, but we are too afraid to really ask

"Are you all right?"

How to answer would take forever

There is no time to really say, so we say we are OK.

The stage light shines again

The actor recites the same lines.

Pamela Buckley.

Foreword

by Mary Wormell

I first met Shirley when she was a cheerful 18-year-old, working at Bowhill stables near Selkirk. Even though I was 12 years her senior, we got on well and gradually became close friends.

Shirley was the one who persuaded me to take part in the Common Riding as I had always been apprehensive. She assured me it was great fun! So along with Sandra Statham (now Smith-Maxwell), Claire Webster and Shirley, I rode the marches—and she was right: I loved it.

We used to meet regularly throughout the summer and go on long hacks together across the hills, or through the woods. I really miss those times. Shirley always seemed to have a new supply of jokes, so we spent most of our time laughing.

When Shirley became ill, it was such a shock to everyone. She was so young and full of life. Throughout her illness, she amazed everyone with her strength of character. She made it easy for anyone who came to visit her as she was open and straight about her condition. But she didn't dwell on it, preferring to talk about more mundane things.

When she was able, we still met up for our rides and Shirley was the same as ever, full of jokes and making us laugh all the way.

After she had been ill for quite a while, and was obviously a lot weaker and thinner than she used to be, I remember asking how she was getting on with her treatment. She told me it was just a matter of time: her body couldn't take any more chemotherapy. I was shocked . . . I'd just never let myself believe that she wasn't going to make it. Shirley was so brave and matter-of-fact, and in the next breath she was telling another joke or funny episode that she'd heard.

I know she spent many days crying and feeling desperate, but she was so keen to be "normal" when she was out and about that we just carried on the same as before, and made the most of the time she had left.

This book is a lovely tribute to Shirley, who was a really good friend to me. I think of her every day and I'll miss her always.

Mary Wornell

Chapter One:

HAPPIER TIMES

S hirley was born at 9:20 am on 19th January 1971—a Tuesday morning—at Selkirk Cottage Hospital. Even then I suppose she was a very lucky baby, because my wife Kath almost lost her six months into the pregnancy. That in itself was a traumatic time—we were living at Langshaw Farm then and Kath awoke one morning to say something was wrong and had to be rushed to hospital in Edinburgh by ambulance, its blue light flashing all the way. At that time I did not have a car and you really find out who your friends are when you have to borrow one to make trips to and from hospital. I will always be grateful to George Alexander for helping us in that way in our hour of need.

On leaving the hospital Kath was told she would have to be very careful for the rest of her pregnancy, but with God's help Shirley made it safely into this world. She was a bonny baby, and despite being the double of her mum, I still failed to pick her out from four babies in the ward at the time, and gave everyone a good laugh as a result.

Our first home was in Bannerfield, a housing scheme in Selkirk, where we lived happily for three years. But in our hearts we always wanted to live in the country, away from town life. By chance I was working on the outskirts of Selkirk, laying concrete floors in the farmer's new shed at Lindean. Chatting to him one day, I explained I was looking for a house in the country and he offered us a cottage which had been standing empty for some time.

Kath and I had looked at this cottage before we were married and had dreamed of living in it. When I told her she couldn't quite believe it, but it was true. We arranged to go and see the cottage that night and knew almost immediately that we would spend the next few years of our lives there.

The transition from town to country life was fantastic, and Kath and Shirley really loved it. One of its most endearing features was there were virtually no worries about traffic, which to Kath and I was a great relief.

Shirley's life—like ours—was one big adventure now, with us buying young chicks, ducks, and geese, and fresh eggs regularly on the menu. Shirley was about three or four before she saw her first pony—Prince, a black fell pony which she shared with her cousin Grace. He was much too big for her, of course, but it was nice to see her sitting up there on the pony's back with her mum.

The years passed and soon it was time for Shirley to start school at Knowepark Primary. I will always remember the way she looked in her nice new school dress—it was a joy to see. Unfortunately, not long after she started, Shirley had two black-outs—one at school and the other in the shop nearby. (Shirley had shown a few early signs of illness when she was only two—her mum sometimes caught her staring blankly into space but at the time we did not take any notice). We took her up to the Sick Children's Hospital in Edinburgh for tests—a frightening experience for Shirley as a young child, and for us as parents, because we were also quite young. There were several wires leading from her head into large machines, in an attempt to trace the cause of the black-outs. Eventually Shirley was diagnosed as epileptic but the doctors said she would probably grow out of it and put her on drugs to control the symptoms.

We thought epilepsy would limit what Shirley could do in terms of horse-riding, but I suppose the writing was on the wall as to how tough our young lass would turn out to be. She always took her pills—sometimes enquiring as to the reason why, but accepting our explanaton that if she missed taking them at certain times of the day, she might fall over and hurt herself.

Shirley was now six or seven, and was pushing her pram around Lindean with Sooty the cat on top and her puppy Sweep on the bottom. By this time Kath had introduced her to Dryden riding centre, where Jenny Macaulay ran classes for all age groups. Kath would pick Shirley up from school, park in a lay-by to allow her to change into her riding gear, and take her straight to riding class. Years later, Kath and Shirley would laugh about the way Shirley had managed to squeeze into her jodhpurs and other riding clothes, eat a roll and drink a can of juice at the same time!

Her very first ride at Dryden was on a pony called Coco and she loved him dearly. This early experience, and tuition from Jenny, gave her the confidence to go on and ride larger horses.

Shirley's second pony was Beauty, a small eleven two hand, with whom Kath taught Shirley to ride over jumps and small fences at weekends.

Life at Lindean was fantastic in those days—as Shirley herself would write later on in life—because all her little friends from school used to come down at nights, weekends, and the long hot summers. The farm at the time was like an adventure playground to children of their age (not the ideal place for them to play, I hasten to add!)

But in 1980 the recession began to bite. The building trade was affected and soon I was unemployed. Strangely enough, it would turn out to be a blessing in disguise because during a really cold snap in January, I approached the farmer, who was having some difficulty in starting up his machinery to feed his animals. I offered him my services straight away and was so successful I was offered a job on the farm. Call it fate or what you will, but I was still working there eight years later.

Working for the farmer, Anthony Aglen, meant I could get grazing from him and perhaps even manage to build Shirley's first stable, feed and hay store. And that's exactly what happened. Shirley had always dreamed of having her own stable at the bottom of the garden, so she could look out of her bedroom window last thing, and say goodnight to her pony. With my new job I was able to give her all these things, and it gave me enormous pleasure to see her face as we built the boxes, haystore and tackroom.

The first pony Shirley would own was Birchie. Kath must have been some wheeler dealer at the time as he was an expensive pony, still in his prime, but she was determined he would be the one for Shirley.

Come rain, hail or shine, Shirley was always determined not to miss the Selkirk Common Riding, the biggest horse event in her calendar—held even more dearly by her than Christmas, I think! The look on her face when she came riding in at the Toll, at the end of the annual 13-mile ride was something to see—and definitely worth all the effort we had made in looking after Birchie, and the expense of feed, transport and vets' bills.

Just like any other youngster her age, Shirley would go to birthday parties but as soon as she got home, off came the nice party dress and on went the jeans so she could go down to the bottom of the garden and do some serious mucking out.

Animals surrounded Shirley all her young life. Once when I was feeding a young calf and her mother in a cattle box, Shirley somehow followed me in without me noticing. When I popped out to fetch a bale of straw for bedding, I was shocked to see Shirley tearing out the door with the cow in hot pursuit. I think she must have come too close to the calf for comfort—so there was a lesson for both of us that day.

One of the farm dogs, Peg, was to be another love of Shirley's. Long retired, Peg spent most of her time tied up at her kennel and was walked just whenever there was time. Shirley asked me to find out whether she could perhaps take Peg for a walk now and again. Happily the farmer was only too pleased to relinquish one of his many chores and soon the two of them became inseparable, Peg spending more time in our house than in her kennel.

One day I noticed that tears were streaming down Shirley's cheeks as she took Peg back to her kennel. She told me she was heartbroken every time she had to do this. The farmer said he saw no reason why Peg—who was starting to look her age—should not have some comfort in her later years and staying with us would probably do her a lot of good. Shirley was delighted when she heard that Peg would join our family.

They were some team—Shirley, Peg, Sweep and Sooty the cat, but she was so happy and that was all that mattered. Whenever she went riding they all set off together, following close behind Birchie.

By this time Kath and Shirley convinced me I should learn to ride, so I started going to Dryden. The idea was that the three of us should ride the marches together, as a family, so I went ahead and hired a horse a week before the Common Riding. One beautiful evening in June Shirley and I went off into the hills around Lindean on our mounts. We were riding along the side of a slippy field and I was in front when my horse either stumbled or slipped, and the next thing I knew I was lying on the ground with a bruised and bleeding nose. As I picked myself up, Shirley turned purple with laughter. I could not blame her, I suppose, as I must have looked a proper sight. Climbing back onto my horse, I asked her what she found so funny and this made her laugh even more. We rode the marches that year, an experience I would not have missed for the world.

By now Shirley was competing at the Yarrow Show, a local agricultural event where anyone with a horse or pony can compete for cups or rosettes, or just generally show off their riding skills. Shirley won many a rosette or small cup on Birchie at such shows, and by the time she was 11 or 12 she was starting to think about cross country events.

At Dryden her instructor Tutti noticed that her new pony Blair and Shirley seemed to click. Even though he was very strong she seemed to push all the right buttons. Other pupils had attempted to win on Blair, but success at competitions was rare unless Tutti rode him. With this in mind, Tutti started to groom Shirley for cross country events. One of her first wins on Blair was at a small country competition at Nether Whitlaw on the outskirts of Selkirk. Shirley was so proud that her rosette took pride of place on the kitchen wall at home.

Shirley went on to shine with Blair at bigger events, including a one-day competition at Oxnam Row, a farm near Jedburgh. This time there was dressage, a cross country course and showjumping all on one day, an event which attracted a wide range of pony clubs from many areas. Shirley came second that day and it was one of the proudest moments of Kath's life when she went up to collect her prize.

By the time Shirley was 15 or 16 she was enjoying going out with her friends and often danced the night away at the rugby club under age disco.

There was one incident I recall during Shirley's teenage years which demonstrated her courage. Two little boys had been playing with matches in the hay shed at Lindean, starting a terrible fire. Only Shirley's quick thinking saved Birchie's life and that of another three or four horses. I was not there at the time, but an eye-witness told me our lass had been very brave, leading the horses past the blazing buildings to safety.

In January we received devastating news about our cottage. The farmer told us he would have to put it up for sale as, unbeknown to us, he was hitting hard times. He had waited until after Christmas to tell us so as not to spoil things, but that did not lessen the blow. I will never forget the look on Kath's face when I revealed the dreadful news to her. At first Shirley did not understand the implications but I had to explain that her stable, tackroom, etc were all at risk and would also be sold off with the cottage.

We were shell-shocked to say the least, having to face the prospect of looking for another house which might be miles from Selkirk and, worse still, far away from Birchie. To our disappointment we ended up moving to another housing scheme in Selkirk, away from the country life we loved and had become accustomed to, with none of the privacy we had taken for granted. We tried very hard and stuck it out for six months, but the call of the country was so strong that we uprooted everything once again and moved to a farm cottage on the south side of the town.

I still had my job at Lindean, however, and Shirley's pony Birch was stabled in the steading alongside all the other horses. It was heart-rending to watch someone else living in our old cottage and using Birchie's old stable.

Around the time Shirley was of school leaving age, a chance to move to a larger house back in Selkirk arose. We grabbed it because the house stood on its own grounds surrounded by a large wall, affording us privacy once again.

Living in the town was very different for Shirley, because all her friends used to walk round town one way, have a cup of coffee or juice, then walk all round town the other way. Although Shirley did it a couple of times, she said it wasn't really her kind of thing and she stopped it.

After leaving school, Shirley started working with a large textile company, Dawson International, and attended college in Galashiels twice each week. Life was to become quite difficult for her as a maturing teenager because she did take umbrage when I laid down the law about the times she was expected to come home from her nights out. Discos, night clubs and dances were all a big part of her life (as it should have been) and I suppose, looking back, the 12 o'clock deadline I imposed was a bit harsh. But she was my only daughter—and a beautiful one at that—and I felt it was right.

When Shirley turned 18, she was offered the chance of a job at the Bowhill riding centre by her friend, Sandra Statham. She would be back beside her beloved horses, so unsurprisingly she accepted. The job entailed mucking out ten or 11 boxes every day and Shirley was in her element, up to her neck in horse dung, then taking out a string of horses round the hills of the estate with her new dog Skippy following close behind.

A flat went with the job but Shirley always phoned her mum every day to let her know what was happening. She popped in to see us regularly, especially on a Saturday, when she would show her mum the new clothes she had bought to wear that evening. On Thursdays she would join her mum so they could both shop for groceries and they would have good laughs together.

Shirley's first real relationship was with a boy called Keith, who was to move into her flat. I had problems coming to terms with this, even though they had been going together for some time. With hindsight, I suppose it was the done thing then, but to a father it was a severe blow. I had big expectations for Shirley because we wanted to give her all the nice things her mum and I could never afford, but in the end I accepted Keith. Shirley loved him dearly and I went on to find out just how nice a young chap he really was.

Shirley's boss Sandra kindly loaned her car for weekly message runs but as the builders' merchants business my partner and I had started was now ticking along nicely, Kath and I decided it was time Shirley should have her first car. This was the chance I had been waiting for—to better myself and hopefully make life a little easier for my family.

Like most teenagers, Shirley enjoyed her job and her social life, but her love of her new-found freedom—and her horses—meant that her relationship with Keith was not going to go much further. He was also heavily into his own hobbies, including cycling and motorbiking. They slowly drifted apart and Shirley ended up living alone again in her flat with her beloved dog Skippy.

By this time Kath and I were living at Sunderland Hall, back in the countryside we loved. It was 1992 and Christmas was coming—but looking back there was never to be another like this one for our family. At the meal Kath noticed that Shirley was not eating very much and looked a little off colour. Christmas and New Year came and went, but Kath was still concerned and made a doctor's appointment for Shirley.

The doctor gave Shirley some pills, putting it down to "boyfriend trouble" and how a young girl might feel, but Kath was astonished to hear this prognosis. After spending an evening with Shirley at the flat, Kath informed me on her arrival home that she was going to seek a second opinion.

The second doctor could see nothing apparently wrong, but decided to take a blood sample, just in case she had missed something . . .

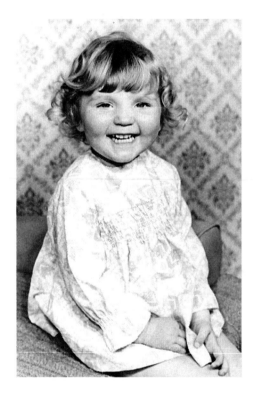

Early smiles and a hint of a mischievous sense of humour from
Shirley at two years of age

Chapter Two:

THE NIGHTMARE BEGINS

Shirley had gone to her GP for a blood test on January 21 and the following day her doctor rang my office to ask how she could contact Shirley as her phone was dead. The previous night had been very stormy and all the lines were down on the Bowhill Estate where Shirley lived and worked as a groom at the riding stables.

I told the doctor she was probably out riding, but if there was a message I would take it up to her later. When the doctor told me they would take a message up and pin it to her door, I knew there was something untoward. No sooner had I returned to my desk after lunch than Shirley called from our home telephone in floods of tears. The note said she must immediately attend Borders General Hospital as there was an abnormality in her blood tests.

I immediately rang Kath at her work to explain what Shirley had told me, and that she was very frightened about the urgent visit to hospital. We met up at the BGH soon afterwards, to find that Shirley had had both head and chest X-rays. One was to look for a tumour, which would explain the sore heads, although at that time there was a local meningitis scare amongst teenagers—indeed a 19-year-old boy had already died from the disease. It was frightening to think Shirley could be in danger from something like that. Chest X-rays had also been taken because Shirley had complained of pains there, and at that point Kath wondered if she had popped a rib falling off her horse, and never noticed.

Unfortunately the X-ray revealed a large dark shadow right in the centre of her chest. By now things were becoming very confused and scary. I knew by the looks on the faces of both Shirley and her mum when I entered the ward that they were looking for answers—from me, somebody, anybody.

Shirley spent one night in the BGH, before being transferred to the Western General Hospital in Edinburgh. Because of her head pain we were sent to the neurological ward, where the tests began in earnest.

The first involved a lumbar puncture—a very painful experience, not just because of the sensitive area in which the needle is inserted, but because the recipient is left with a blinding headache afterwards. That's when I began to realise how much pain my daughter was really in. It meant she had no appetite, although she was probably frightened too.

Shirley looked so helpless last thing that day before we set off home for Selkirk. On the way back we discussed how no-one was really telling us anything for definite, but resolved to keep thinking positively for Shirley's sake.

I could not fail to notice the strain on Kath's face—she and Shirley had always been so very close.

As nothing positive was found in Shirley's head they transferred her to the respiratory ward. It was only about three days into the tests but she was looking frail and thin through not eating. I was now becoming very worried about her.

The ward she was admitted to had an old woman in the next bed who was dying and that alone was frightening enough. We were now in a different world, far away from the horses and stables which had been a normal part of every day life for Shirley only 72 hours ago.

By this time we were at the hospital at 8:30 am and staying until 11:30 pm. Most of our day was spent trying to persuade Shirley to eat something, anything. I then realised how much I loved that frail little girl lying there, crying and terrified of what they were going to do to her next. Throughout her teenage years we had had what you might call a "love-hate" relationship because I was fairly strict, but I had always loved her and had never shown it till now. All I wanted to do as I sat by the bedside was to enfold her in a big reassuring hug, but I settled instead for holding hands. I had to leave the ward on several occasions because it was difficult to control my emotions and I could not let Shirley see how distraught I was feeling.

The doctors were now sticking needles into Shirley's neck for a biopsy so they could establish what we were up against. At the end of the first week they decided to remove a piece of the offending mass inside her chest, using a giant needle attached to a large mechanised arm. They used a local anaesthetic, but it was horrendous for Shirley to see this happening. We sat outside the room and when they eventually wheeled her out on her bed I had never seen anyone so frightened in my life. A vein in her neck was pulsating so violently it looked as if it was about to burst. She was crying and I felt so helpless, but I knew I had to remain strong. However, that night Kath and I cried nearly all the way home.

By now Kath's brother Mike and my family—especially my sister Mary—were mucking in and helping us, feeding the dogs, and making us hot cups of tea when we came home.

The next day was scary because when Kath took Shirley to the toilet she collapsed on the floor through a combination of weakness and fear. That night Shirley told us she had had an out-of-body experience in which she had floated up to the corner of the room and looked down from the ceiling on herself in bed, with us at her bedside. She also said she had seen Granny (Kath's mum) who had died six years ago.

I was by now demented with worry and although we had our suspicions, there was still no clear indication as to what the problem was. Shirley was now down to seven stone from nine stone seven and looked very weak. I was determined to pin someone down and was devastated when a lady consultant revealed—off the record—that they were looking for a tumour, which might be malignant. It was a complete bombshell which left me shaking in my boots.

I pretended to go back to the car for a cup of tea with Kath but was barely able to contain myself on the way out. We sat in the car, with the rain pouring down outside, and after telling her what I had been told we just burst into tears and sobbed uncontrollably. I felt I was at the lowest point in the whole chain of events and on reflection, it was probably the bleakest day in my life. Ten years ago I had been at my mother's bedside when she died, and that night the grief I felt was something I thought could never be repeated again in my lifetime. Now my only daughter had a life-threatening illness but it was so much worse because she was part of Kath and I.

After leaving the hospital at night, I would usually phone my sister Evelyn, who would in turn keep the family informed. That bleak night, I remember telling her the devastating news we had received, with me sobbing in a way I have never done since I was a boy, and Kath breaking her heart in the sitting room next door. I was so upset I could not get the words out so Evelyn told me to break off and call back the next day.

Back at the hospital the doctors said the tests had been inconclusive, and the next plan was to send Shirley across to the City Hospital for a biopsy, which meant removing a gland in her chest for further pathology tests. She was now so afraid but all we could do was keep reassuring her that everything would be all right.

I should say at this point that the nurses and doctors who helped us were exceptional in the care they provided—especially in the little extra gestures, such as providing beds for us, because Shirley wanted us to be with her all the time.

We were with her when she received her pre-med and lying there unconscious she looked like a fourteen-year-old. We sat in a small waiting room during the two-and-a-half hour operation pondering on what they might find. Shirley emerged from theatre with an oxygen mask and several tubes attached to different parts of her body. When she came round, she started to cry, which meant us having to choke back the tears. We had to leave her to recover that day, but before we went I sought out the surgeon, who said the operation had been a success and that a piece of the gland would have to be tested by three different pathologists before a full diagnosis could be made. To our astonishment the result came back within hours.

We now knew what we were up against. Shirley had lymphoma, a form of cancer. The dreaded word had now been spoken out loud, and it was a bombshell to the three of us. The doctor explained that out of more than 250 different cancers, Shirley's was the 'preferable' one to have because hers was curable with the correct treatment. Fortunately she was being treated by someone eminent in his field, Dr. Robert Leonard. At our first meeting he did not pull any punches because he stated clearly that he was not going for treatment but a cure: chemotherapy would get under way immediately.

It was horrendous to watch the specialist nurses trying to raise a vein in Shirley's hand because she was so thin. We were told there would be hair loss with the treatment, which especially worried her as a young girl conscious of her appearance.

Kath and I cried on the way home, with the devastating news beginning to take its toll. An event like this puts life into perspective, and I called my partner when I got home to tell him that my business and everything else was now secondary to Shirley's illness.

Treatment continued the next day in tablet form, which caused her to become very sick and nauseous. It lasted from Monday until Thursday and she appeared to rally round for the weekend, before the process was repeated. This was the pattern for the next few weeks, by which time Shirley's hair had become thin and straggly. It was then she decided to have it cut short.

Life at home had to go on, with Kath and I working whenever we could. Sometimes I would pop in to make a meal for Shirley—if I could persuade her to eat anything. It was with a heavy heart that I would leave her after those visits, lying in bed at Sunderland Hall farmhouse looking like someone from a concentration camp.

I was now losing faith, thinking that Shirley might never recover from what could be a long illness. But I always gave myself a kick, knowing I must stay strong because she would need all the support we could give. The tears flowed more readily now whenever I was on my own, and my family's plight overshadowed everything. Some nights I would attempt to go into Selkirk for a drink but return a short while later, having never had the courage to go into a pub in case someone asked me about Shirley.

Because of the difficulty in getting veins raised on Shirley's arm, she now had a Hickman line to administer drugs into her body. It was a small operation but a scary experience for Shirley, although it definitely made life easier in terms of getting blood samples, etc. The line had to be cleaned once a week with special drugs and on one occasion there must have been bacteria lurking in the line because when it was flushed out Shirley was hit by an infection. Within half an hour she was very ill with a raging temperature, and had to have antibiotics round the clock for four days, before she was well enough to come home. Sometimes when I brought Shirley home from hospital she was so weak I had to practically carry her to the car.

As the weeks went by the treatment entered a new phase, with chemo being pumped in four days at a time. Dr. Leonard had stepped things up because Shirley had stopped responding to her treatment. Once she became really ill with a raging temperature and to our shock we discovered she had pneumonia. All her previous bouts were nothing compared to what she was enduring now. I have never seen anybody so violently sick: it was coming straight from the lung, according to nursing staff.

Shirley was very concerned about being sick in front of me as I have always had a hang-up about seeing people doing this. However, I must have drawn strength from somewhere because I was OK holding her head over the bowl. It's different when your own child is being ill.

Nine months had passed and the illness was taking its toll. Indeed Shirley was now talking about giving up because of her horrendous treatment. Although it was easy for us to say, Kath and I told her there was no alternative but to plug away, and we set a target for her to be on the road to recovery by Christmas.

My work was suffering now as I could not fully concentrate on the daily round of tasks which the business demanded. I did what I could, but I told Shirley that no matter where I was, or whatever I was doing, all she had to do was get a message to me and I would respond right away.

It was a great treat to have Shirley home with us for Christmas because if she had been in hospital we would have had nothing to celebrate.

In January 1994, Shirley went into remission and was starting to look her old self again—a beautiful young girl any father would be proud of. We were now going for monthly checks and praying the traumas of the past were well and truly behind us. I was drinking every night to try and help me sleep but decided to stop. Kath had started smoking again but promised she would stop too.

Our hopes were soon dashed. In April Shirley's disease returned with a vengeance, requiring more intensive chemotherapy. Lumps had appeared on her groin, neck, armpits and lung. Before we went to hospital, Kath and I decided to have a quiet word with Dr. Leonard as to the seriousness of the illness, and to find out what we were up against now.

The doctor was frank with me from the word go, giving me the news I had been dreading: the disease was now much more advanced and Shirley only had a 10 per cent chance of survival. He also said the chemotherapy was more or less just to slow it down and a cure looked very doubtful. I didn't know what to do with this knowledge but we had to know—there was no sense burying our heads in the sand. If she was to become unresponsive to treatment, Dr. Leonard explained, her time with us could be as little as one or two months. She was released and sent home with morphine amongst her medication.

Kath and I were devastated.

Why Shirley, I wondered angrily, of all people, after all the problems she had had in life—epilepsy, birth marks on her legs—all big things to a young girl. We decided there and then not to admit defeat and just soldier on regardless. But we were hoping for a miracle now.

Because I could not fully take in all that our consultant had told us, I made an appointment to see our family doctor in Selkirk. He was quite shocked to learn of Shirley's possible fate. But we all agreed not to tell her how poorly she actually was.

It was not long before her condition worsened still further, with Shirley now having great difficulty in swallowing. Kath was always near to give pain killers and comfort her through the blackest moments of dispair. It was a blessing to witness this special care I believe only a mother can give her child.

Shirley was under the impression that after another two or three treatments, she would receive a "big blast" of chemo. She and I spoke well into the night about the forthcoming Selkirk Common Riding, her special time of the year, telling me just how much she loved it but being so ill she decided she did not mind missing it this year as there would be plenty others. Little did the poor lass know how ill she was.

Whenever Shirley was released from hospital her blood count dropped, and we had to be extremely careful as a common cold could develop into something life threatening.

At certain times after treatment, the doctor had to come in and take samples, which I hurriedly whisked away to hospital for analysis. The results were then telephoned to the Western General in Edinburgh, to allow them to keep a close watch on Shirley's condition.

Michael and Sal Strang Steel, who had had to employ someone else to do Shirley's job, were especially kind, refusing to take any rent for her flat throughout her illness. They promised Shirley that as soon as she was fit enough she could take Lady Strang Steel's hunter James for a hack. Things like this kept Shirley really focused on getting better.

However, her health deteriorated yet again and the doctor decided she would have to return to hospital the next day. When hearing that Shirley was en route, one of the staff nurses, Evelyn Telfer, who had looked after her so dedicatedly over the past year, immediately gave up her lunch break and waited for the ambulance to arrive.

Evelyn and another nurse, Fiona, were to become Shirley's very good friends. On one occasion Fiona called up Lothian and Borders Police HQ which is close to the hospital and arranged a visit to the police stables and dog kennel as a "pick me up" for Shirley. What a grand tonic it was for her to be back beside her beloved horses, albeit briefly, because she was still beaming when her mum and I arrived later.

Unfortunately nothing would stay in Shirley's stomach now, not even epanutin, the drug which controlled her epilepsy. It was discovered that her red cell count was extremely low and she had caught another infection. She was also bleeding from her stomach into her bowels. The answer was an immediate blood transfusion and antibiotics, and all liquids over the next two days went into her body by IV. Because her haemoglobin was also low, her blood was not clotting well and she suffered nose bleeds for two days. Our Shirley never moaned or complained and was more concerned about how her mother and I felt, especially if the scarf round her head slipped and revealed her bare head.

Kath and I were like ships passing in the night and were both exhausted but it was difficult for us to sleep when we were so worried. Through all this Shirley was more worried about how we were coping and she was some corker, actually winking to us through all that pain and suffering. Thankfully, with the skilled help of the doctors and nurses, she started improving yet again.

On May 18 the doctors sent a tiny exploratory camera down into Shirley's stomach to try and find out where the bleeding was coming from. They thought perhaps that she had an ulcer from all the retching, or from the disease itself.

Shirley was now on a morphine drip attached to her arm, which injected drugs automatically at set intervals. She was now showing the hospital what a fighter she was, and I thought that anyone faced with a similar situation could learn from Shirley's approach that when everything looks really bleak, it's time to batten down the hatches in order to fight another day.

She told Kath that she looked to me for a lot of support now, which felt really good as I had not always been there for her during her teenage years. Here I was getting a second chance to make amends for laying down the law and I was very grateful.

At this stage we were taking things one step at a time. People were so kind, asking us about Shirley all the time, and it was a great tonic to know that others were thinking about us because we often felt lonely.

It may be hard to believe but on May 28 we discovered that Shirley had asked Dr. Leonard whether it was possible for her not to have any more harsh treatment before the Common Riding in June, as it would leave her free of sickness and allow her to ride. Dr. Leonard okayed this but insisted on seeing her a few days before the ride to check her health. He told us that her body had been so racked by chemo over the past year that even if she needed more treatment, she would not have been able to accept any. We were also worried to find out that her Hickman line was to be removed, because that was the way Shirley's drugs were administered to her.

Dr. Leonard said Shirley was being allowed to ride because her immune system was holding the disease at bay, but at the first signs of sweats, lumps or bumps, he was to be notified right away. He also told her to have a jolly good Common Riding.

Now here was a girl who had been so ill just days before, planning to ride 13 miles over hills and moors, over ditches and burns—an event that challenges even fit people. But that did not worry Shirley: she was more concerned about not being allowed to take James round the marches.

The big day arrived and Shirley, with the help of her mum, washed, groomed and cleaned James. She was so thin we had to make her a bumnah, a piece of sheepskin sewn to the top of her saddle to make the ride more bearable.

I borrowed a camcorder to film the whole event and it was utterly fantastic to see our daughter smiling again. Kath and I had tears in our eyes when we saw her come in at the Toll—the end of the ride—and she received huge cheers from the thousands of people gathered there.

But the smiles were short lived because on the Sunday, Shirley told us the sweats, lumps and bumps were back again. When we told Dr. Leonard he was surprised the symptoms had returned so quickly. He told us with deep regret that if she responded to future treatment she would probably live for another one or two years at most. If she was to become unresponsive to treatment, her time with us could be as little as two months. Kath and I were devastated but we decided there and then not to admit defeat and just soldier on regardless. We were hoping for a miracle.

I had read about a faith healer in The Sunday Post called Finbar Nolan, the seventh son of a seventh son who lived in Dublin and was much acclaimed by his fellow countrymen. I phoned his home and spoke to his wife who said he was working in the west of Ireland, but when I explained the situation to her, and how ill our daughter was, she asked if Shirley could travel and I said she could at that moment. When I spoke to Finbar himself on his return later that week, I gave him Shirley's prognosis and explained that time was running out. We arranged to meet in Ireland the following week and arrived at Dublin airport on June 30, 1994.

At our meeting, Finbar said he would have to see Shirley on three consecutive days, although we had planned to be in Ireland for only two. I had to try and change our flight times and was at first horrified to learn that we would have to pay almost a whole fare to do so—especially as we were not terribly well off at the time. But when I explained that we were in their country to see a faith healer, the airline immediately allowed us to pay just £90, and wished us all the best in our endeavours to find a cure for Shirley. I must say that in general the people of Ireland were kindness itself and Kath and I will never forget them for helping us in our hour of need.

After Shirley's second visit, she felt fine when she went for her appointment but on arriving back at our rooms she felt terrible, as though she had just had a bout of chemo. She was also feeling sick, which was strange. This raised our hopes that at long last something was actually working, but we did not read too much into it, in case there was more disappointment looming ahead. If it did not work, the alternative was unthinkable.

At this time Ireland were playing in the World Cup and doing very well under the auspices of the great Bobby Charlton. Much to Kath's dismay Shirley asked if I would take her out to the pub one night to sample the atmosphere as all the streets were bedecked with Irish flags. We were no sooner in one establishment when Shirley got involved in a long and protracted conversation with a girl of her own age. They were speaking about horses, of course, and believe it or not, the girl did the same job as Shirley, so they had much in common. It was gratifying to see her looking so happy—a first, I can tell you, for a while.

We arrived back home and things just seemed to come and go. Shirley was able to go on holiday with her friend Janet, a break she enjoyed and truly deserved. Her return visits to the Oncology Department at the Western continued and there was never a dull moment on the journey, as Shirley related some of the antics they had been up to.

Shirley now had terrible pains in her leg and was taking ten painkillers a day to try and ease them. This was due to a gland problem, so it meant chemo yet again—this time in pill form. It was devastating to watch her lose all her hair yet again.

But this seemed to make no difference to a young man who was becoming known to us. David Lowthian was four years Shirley's junior but was mature for his age, which he would prove to us later in more difficult times.

Being fiercely independent, Shirley was still living on her own: I think she did not want anyone to think she was "giving in" to the disease. Fortunately David was doing little jobs for her, like bringing up coal and logs from the cellar, tasks she was now too weak to do herself.

It must have been very difficult for a young girl to try and lead a normal life in such circumstances, but try she did and she soon began to fall in love with David. The wonderful thing, as Kath once commented, was that he fell in love with her when she felt so 'unlovely'; when she had not a single hair on her head. He simply loved the person he saw—her personality and great sense of humour.

Another reason that Shirley kept going was that friends gave her their horses to ride, putting a bit of normality back into her life.

It was now December 1994 and Shirley and David were very much in love, although they had to face problems not normally associated with a couple so young. David was taking on a lot with Shirley's medical—and now some psychological—problems. We had been warned that she might be affected psychologically when we first encountered this awful disease. Because she was feeling ugly and thin, she often felt jealous and her mind sometimes ran wild with silly notions. At one point she would not even watch television as she could not bear to watch anyone glamorous. Fortunately, she was able to see a psychologist, which she said made her feel so much better because she could speak to someone outside the family about her problems.

Her condition was now severe, with pains in her back and swollen leg requiring her to take 20mgs of oral morphine. Every journey to Edinburgh involved packing a little bag with all her medication.

Christmas 1994 came and went, Shirley describing it in her diary as "fun although a bit of an anti-climax . . . but it was nice to be with mum and dad, and I think we had more to celebrate than most families this year." But she was concerned that her Mum, Dad and David would be beside themselves with worry when they heard her screaming in agony in her room because of the pain.

At that stage we promised to buy Shirley a car, believing it would help her take her mind off some of her problems. She told us she would love either a Peugeot 205 or a Golf turbo diesel, so we scoured the countryside for both, but after much ado the car she eventually settled for was a Fiat Tipo.

Meanwhile, the illness continued to take its toll, plaguing Shirley with a terrible itch causing her to scratch her legs and feet so severely they bled. No ointment could relieve the itch as it was in her bloodstream, a side of effect of the disease, and it was particularly bad at night.

In February 1995 I read about George Fox, a Lanarkshire minister who, to my amazement, was performing faith healing at his church. I hastily made an appointment for a week's time, although Shirley was feeling pretty low and would take some persuading to go. David, Kath, Shirley and I met him and watched as he laid on hands, and told Shirley just before she left that she would feel very tired for about 15 minutes on the way home. Incredibly, no sooner had we set off than she curled up in a little ball on the seat and fell soundly asleep for about that length of time. When she awoke, we just looked at each other in amazement, wondering if this was the remedy that was going to work.

Although Shirley had been prescribed anti-sickness pills, often this did not help when she had chemotherapy. Once again her blood count was low and her Selkirk GP wanted her to go back into hospital for a transfusion. She was in more pain and an X-ray revealed the disease had spread to the remaining good lung. We promised Shirley we would bring her back home as soon as she felt well again.

Shirley became so desperate not to go back to hospital that she promised the doctors she would take their special injections, one in the morning and one at night, as an outpatient. Luckily she and David were living with us at the time, so we could keep an eye on her increasingly precarious state of health. Sometimes even oral morphine could not combat her pain, and on several occasions she had to call out the doctor to give her a strong injection. Although she was seeing a hypnotherapist now and it appeared to be doing her some good, she sometimes said she might be better off dead.

Shirley picked herself up once again and managed to ride her beloved James, with her devoted dog Skippy running alongside, but the good times were few and far between now. A lump had appeared on the side of her neck and had swelled so much it had started to cut off the circulation to the side of her face, making her teeth hurt—like having constant toothache.

On one of Shirley's better days in May, 1995, Kath suggested we went for run to the coast on our own. On the way there, Kath broke the news that Shirley and David were planning to become engaged. It was hard to accept with everything else that was going on in my mind: he's only 20 years old, I said—does David really know what he is doing? The hurt on Kath's face was evident because this was meant to be a joyous announcement. I was forced to think again and after the initial hesitation, I decided: why not? Shirley's so ill, we are all so distraught and uptight—if it makes the young ones happy, then we are happy too. No sooner had we begun our walk along the sea front than Kath dropped a further bombshell—Shirley and David wanted to get married! I was worried about the cost because all our money was tied up in our relatively new business, but when Kath looked at me despairingly, I just thought what the hell! With a bit of luck and some help, I was sure we could pull it off.

This was one decision I would never regret and all the way home we spoke about the wedding. If nothing else it took our minds of Shirley's illness, something we had hitherto believed was impossible. By the time we got home we were greeted by two pensive faces, but when we congratulated them on their news, they were delighted, and we promised we would make the wedding happen somehow. We closed the door behind us and as we walked away we heard David exclaiming: "Yes, yes, yes, yes". We both grinned at the prospect of having something to look forward to.

Unfortunately Shirley's radiotherapy treatment was not having the desired effect and the disease was now widespread. It meant more chemo and yet another trip to hospital, with her blood count very low and her temperature high. Over the next few days the impending wedding looked like a forlorn hope.

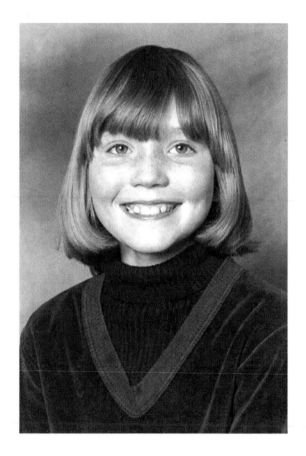

A school photograph of Shirley, taken when she was eight years old.

Chapter Three:

SHIRLEY'S COURAGE

I will never forget the night a consultant at the BGH took it upon himself to have a word with Shirley about her prognosis. Until now I had carried all the knowledge of her illness, and if she wanted to know something, she only had to ask. The doctor told her she was so ill she would only have two or three weeks to live, before the last good part of her lung was affected. Shirley asked what it would be like at "the end" and he explained that a girl of her age with a strong heart might find it difficult to breathe, but she would be under medication and not know a thing.

When I got there, I was distraught to find Shirley crying, and told the consultant he should not have burdened her with the prognosis. He apologised, but explained that she had only weeks to live—news which left me completely shattered. The doctor also said it was difficult for the nurses who were treating Shirley as many of them were just young girls themselves, and it was heartbreaking for them to know what they did.

Panicking, I thought he could have made a mistake; he said he wished he had. He promised to let Shirley home once her temperature was stable, and in the future she could be rushed through casualty, and straight to the ward, to save time.

I returned to Shirley's room, trying to keep up the pretence that I had so expertly managed in the past. The next two hours I spent with her before David returned to the hospital felt like a year.

When I got home, my sister Mary and Kath were talking about the forthcoming wedding but I immediately told them it was off. When Kath and I spoke in private, she was devastated to hear my news. Our first thoughts were for Shirley back at the hospital, but the wedding that had been set for August 19th would have to be postponed, indefinitely.

This latest burden was horrendous: it would be so for any parent. It gave us a sick feeling in our stomachs to think that a child we had nurtured through birth, infancy, childhood and teenage years, would be lost to us in only two or three weeks' time.

Kath immediately asked me to seek a second opinion. I called Dr Leonard in Edinburgh and after disclosing the relevant facts, he agreed with his colleague. This made us feel quite low because all through the treatment Dr Leonard always managed to come up with something—hence Shirley's total faith in him. Sadly for us, there was to be no miracle this time.

When we returned to the hospital, we found David and his mum Evelyn speaking about the impending wedding, and Shirley looking extremely upset. At that time no-one—not even her—knew that we would have to postpone everything. When David and his mum left, Shirley had a bloody good cry.

We tried to keep up her spirits by saying we could perhaps try another form of treatment—chemo, a faith healer, anything. But words could not offer much comfort, and she coped by completely blanking out the conversation she had had with the consultant. We told the doctor the next day that we wanted her back home with us just as soon as she was able.

Two or three days later we brought Shirley home, and it was fantastic to have her in her room again. Although her temperature was quite high, the doctor knew that being home was far more therapeutic than any medicines he could prescribe her in hospital.

After only a week Shirley announced she was getting out of bed, to try and become more mobile. In all honesty, I think she was trying to prove her doctors wrong.

It had been uppermost in my mind to cancel the wedding arrangements—until one Saturday night, when I found Shirley and David sitting on the floor, poring over wedding brochures. When I asked what they were up to, Shirley looked at me with tear-filled, swollen eyes and asked me why I had cancelled their wedding. I told her I hadn't and left the room feeling somewhat bruised. Kath explained that Shirley had not accepted what she had been told and her forthcoming marriage was very dear to her.

That night, frustrated at this new dilemma, I cried myself to sleep. But the next morning I called the family into the sitting room. I put it to them that the wedding could be brought forward a month to July 1st, and with God's help, we might be able to pull it off.

We had a month to organise things, including a wedding dress, the church, a hall for the reception, and wedding cars. After setting a new date, I went to see the minister at Clovenfords, but he was away in France, so I had to ask someone else. Tom Elliot, a local farmer and church elder, could not have been more helpful when I pleaded my case, and after checking the church diary, he reported—to my delight—that the date in question was indeed available.

Shirley and I had often passed the little church at Clovenfords on our way to and from hospital, and had once remarked that it would have been her dream to walk down the aisle on my arm and marry the man of her dreams. Now, fingers crossed, it looked as if the dream might soon become a reality.

A frantic phonecall to the council department responsible for the letting of the Victoria Hall in Selkirk determined that this also was available—it appeared that God was on our side, and looking after us!

We soon became far too busy to dwell on the terrible news about Shirley. She would design her own dress and my sister Mary would make it for her. Laying our hands on the necessary silk fabric was also easy as my partner's wife ran a business buying material. In fact Robert and Miranda generously gave Shirley the material as a wedding present.

The making of the dress was now under way, with Shirley making occasional trips for fitting. The illness had abated slightly during this period, and it was great to see her so excited. Meanwhile, Kath and David's mum Evelyn were busy organising flowers for the church, buttonholes, and finalising the guest list.

Next on the cards was a check-up with Dr Leonard. When Shirley told him of her wedding plans, he immediately congratulated her. She asked him for one last thing: to make sure she would be fit enough to walk down the aisle on her big day and marry her beloved David. To this end, after a thorough examination, Dr Leonard said he would increase her dose of steroids. The drug had probably helped keep Shirley alive over the past few years, but it could not be taken indefinitely because of its serious side effects, such as brittle bones and occasionally kidney failure.

When she got home Shirley started her high dose of steroids which, when they took effect, made her absolutely ravenous. She was now getting up in the middle of the night, eating bacon and eggs, jam sandwiches and crisps, and in only a week she gained a good 12 pounds. By now she was starting to look like her old self again and it was wonderful for her mum and I to see her happy, and looking forward to the wedding.

I had managed to book two large white Rolls Royces for the big day, much to Shirley's delight. The other thing she thought would make the occasion perfect was The Strangers, a band much sought after locally for weddings. One of the songs they performed was "Unchained Melody", a hit for Robson and Jerome at the time, and a firm favourite of Shirley and David's. The band were already booked up, but when we explained the situation to their lead singer, he checked with the people who had originally booked them, and they graciously agreed to cancel, passing on their best wishes to us all.

A couple of days later Shirley had to have a blood transfusion as her levels were so low and she later commented to a number of people that she must have received some of Linford Christie's blood as her energy levels were so good!

All was going well, but the next problem to be surmounted was the fact that Shirley and David wanted to go to Majorca for their honeymoon. The determined bride-to-be had already enquired about the matter of travel for a sick person, as normal insurance was completely out of the question. The race was on to find a company who would cover them in the event of Shirley turning ill abroad.

We also warned her that she might suffer from prickly heat in Spain. By now the itching was back with a vengeance, bringing tears to her eyes and interrupting her sleep. We tried anything to help ease the itch, even putting the likes of frozen peas on her legs and feet, because the ice cubes were melting too quickly and making the bed wet. But Shirley remained determined to go—not for one week but two, which made things even more risky. Kath and I were worried sick at the prospect, and I tried to dissuade them from going for a fortnight, but after being told it might be their last holiday, I backed down. The final obstacle was overcome when my cousin found us a suitable insurance company which would meet the cost of an air ambulance if Shirley turned ill in Majorca.

Shirley and David were thrilled when the local paper, The Selkirk Weekend Advertiser, covered their engagement and had been so delighted with the photographs taken by my cousin, James Rutherford, that they asked him to take the wedding photos. He said he would be delighted to perform the task.

To make sure David knew what a responsibility he was taking on, I met his father Gordon Lowthian to see how he felt about things. He was really quite upset at our meeting and had great difficulty talking about the forthcoming event. All he could think about was the fact that Kath and I were about to lose our daughter to this awful disease. But if they wanted to get married, he would not stand in their way and indeed would do everything in his power to help.

The wedding dress was now nearly complete, and I was assured by both Shirley and Mary that I would be extremely proud to walk down the aisle with my daughter.

The drawing up of the guest list had been a priority task, with the invitations being sent out soon after. Dr. Leonard, along with nurses Evelyn Telfer and Fiona were included on the list: we were glad to provide a different—and so much happier—focus for us all to come together.

The night before the wedding, the bridesmaids, Claire Webster and Lucy Wormell, cracked open a bottle of champagne and it was so good to see Shirley's bright smile again. It fairly radiated round the room, setting the atmosphere for the next day.

It was July 1st at last and everyone was so excited. Shirley was even mentioned on Radio Borders and to top it all she won a bottle of champagne to help her celebrate her big day. When Shirley came out of her room, to say she looked beautiful would be an understatement. I stood there totally gobsmacked and tears were not far away. At 46 years of age I had seen a few weddings in my time, but to have Shirley on my arm looking so beautiful made this the proudest day of my life. It's one I will remember till the day I die.

Kath looked stunning in her red suit and hat, and posed with the bridesmaids for photographs before we set off in the two cars.

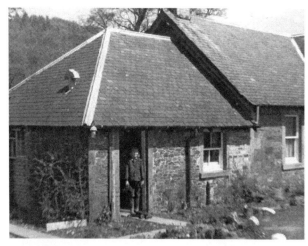

Left: Life in the farm cottage at Lindean was idyllic, far away from the noise and bustle of the town.

Below: Shirley's love affair with horses began at about age four with her pony Prince, which she shared with her cousin Grace.

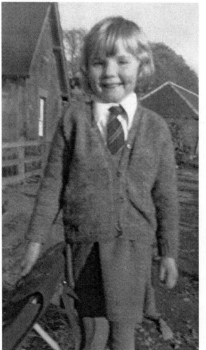

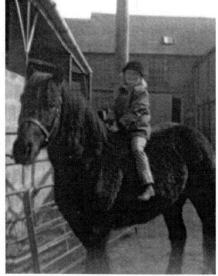

Left: Shirley looking smart for her first day at Knowepark Primary School.

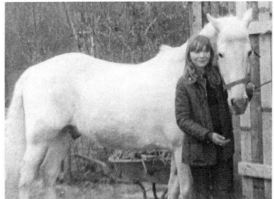

Left: Birchie, the pony bought for Shirley when she was 10 years old. All the effort and expense in keeping him was worth it, according to parents Jim and Kath. Shirley rode Birchie safely round the Selkirk Marches at the Common Riding, 1985

Right: Shirley at the Yarrow Show in 1986. She was blossoming from a quiet schoolgirl into a pretty teenager with a lively sense of fun.

Below: Shirley rides Birchie in at the Toll after a 13-mile ride in the Selkirk Common Riding, 1987. Mum Kath rides Blair (centre), and on the right, on Tam, is Tutti Arres, owner of Dryden Riding Centre.

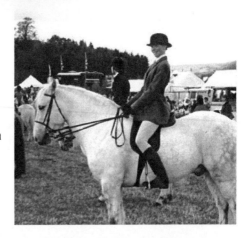

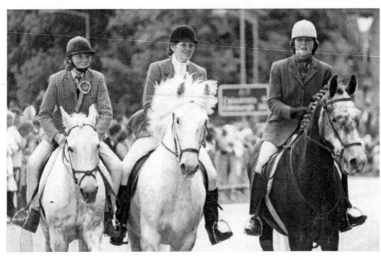

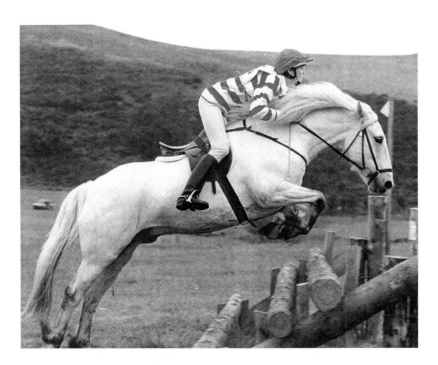

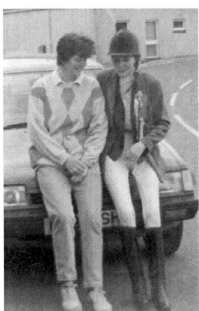

Above: Shirley riding
'Blair' at a competition at
Oxnam Row, Jedburgh,
1990.

Left: In 1995 the illness was taking
its toll but it could not dampen
Shirley's enthusiasm for riding. She
asked for her treatment to be put
on hold to allow her to take part in
that year's Common Riding festival.
Here she shares the experiences of
a memorable day with mum Kath,
outside their home in Selkirk.

Right: Despite Shirley's illness—and her loss of hair—David Lowthian fell in love with the girl underneath all the problems, the shy animal lover with a warm personality and great sense of humour. Several months after they met, they announced their wish to marry. This photograph was taken to celebrate their engagement.

Photos: James Rutherford.

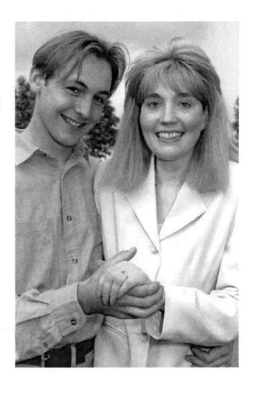

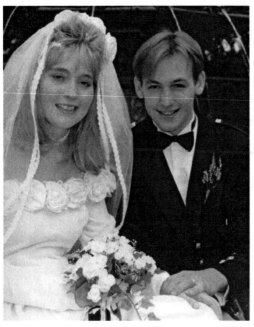

Left: Shirley and David were married at Caddonfoot Parish Church on a sunny day in July, 1995. The bride designed her own wedding dress and was involved in the planning of every aspect of the day, boosted by higher than normal doses of steroids. The couple were married by the Rev. David Kellas.

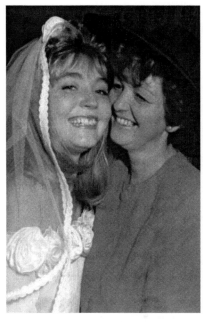

Left: A favourite photo of Shirley's mum Kath, taken at their family home on the morning of the wedding.

Below: Pictured before the bridal party set off for the church are (l to r) bridesmaid Claire Webster, father Jim, Shirley, mum Kath and flower girl Lucy Wormell, then aged 10 years. (Lucy's mother, Mary, wrote the foreword for this book.)

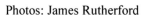

Photos: James Rutherford

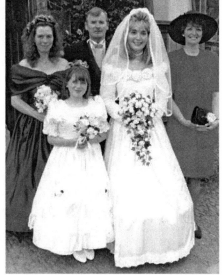

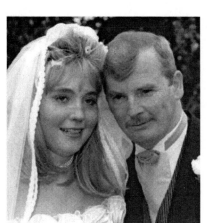

Left: Shirley and father Jim, pictured on their return to the reception in Selkirk. The occasion was emotional but enjoyable—one the family will never forget.

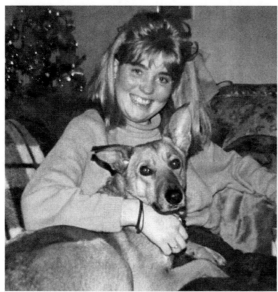

Left: Shirley with her beloved dog Skip. She wanted to live as normal a life as possible and managed many a bright smile when she was out and about. But there were many private moments of despair (below) when she suffered severe bouts of depression and spent many long hours crying as her condition worsened.

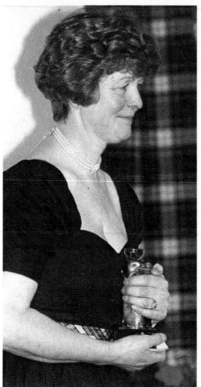

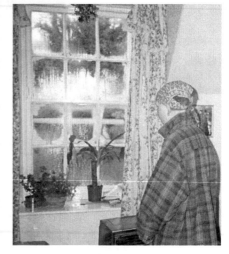

Left: Kath McCallum accepts a 'Great Scot' award on behalf of Shirley. The event was organised by 'The Sunday Mail' and the award, a specially engraved Caithness Crystal ornament in the shape of a thistle, was presented by rugby personality Gavin Hastings.

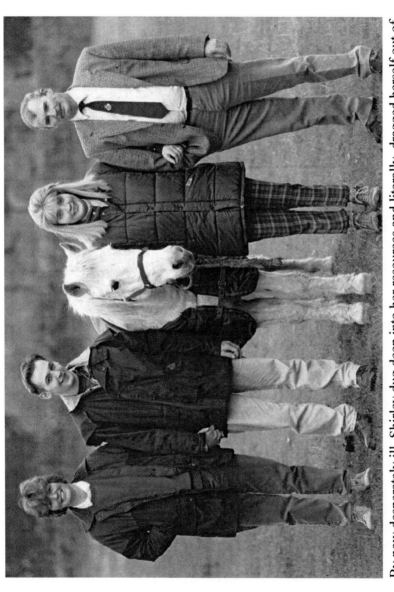

By now desperately ill, Shirley dug deep into her resources and literally dragged herself out of bed to appear in this photo, specially taken for the 'Great Scot' awards. Photo: Courtesy of The Sunday Mail.

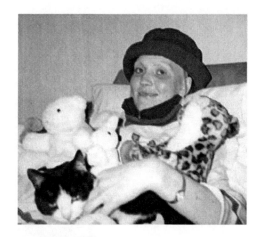

Right: Shirley at home in
Whinfield Road in 1995.

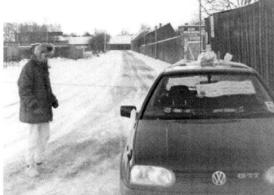

Left: The black Golf
GTI which Jim and
Kath gave to Shirley on
her last Christmas.
Although she had been
excited at the prospect
of owning the car of her
dreams, she actually
was too ill to drive it
herself, apart from on
the odd occasion.

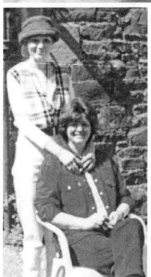

Left: A treasured moment for Shirley with
mum Kath. The two enjoyed a very close
relationship.

Below: A moment of rest for a tired but contented
Shirley, with pup Kalie, in her own flat.

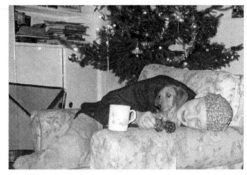

On the way to church, I asked Shirley if she was nervous and she responded by holding my hand. I felt so proud when people looked at us in the car, and as we neared the church I told her there might be a few people waiting outside, but that she shouldn't be nervous. As it happened, it wasn't the bride who was nervous but me!

It was all I could do to contain myself when I handed Shirley over to David at the altar. I nearly cried in front of everyone while singing the hymn, "The Lord's My Shepherd", but a nudge from Kath helped me keep myself together. She said later that if I had lost it she would have started as well. But who could blame us for a shedding a tear or two, when we were watching the wedding of our lovely daughter, who was dying from a horrible disease we were powerless to stop.

The last hymn to be sung, "All Things Bright and Beautiful", completed a perfect ceremony. Everyone present commented on Shirley's dress, saying how beautiful and unusual it was, and how radiant and happy she was looking.

Everyone on the guest list knew the reason for the quick wedding. Some gave David and Shirley money to spend on their honeymoon as they knew that material things would be of little use to them in the near future. As parents, it hurt us to know what lay ahead, but we were determined to make the most of this special day.

In my speech at the reception, I said I would not have given Shirley's hand in marriage lightly to anyone, but I was certain that David was the best. I knew in my heart I was not losing a daughter but gaining a son-in-law.

The newlyweds started off the dancing with their favourite song and they looked quite enchanting together.

In the early hours of the morning, Kath and I reflected on the day's events as we walked home. Although there was a nightmare lurking around the corner, we vowed to take just one day at a time.

We helped Shirley pack, making sure she had all the right medication with her. When they finally set off, they promised to call home at the end of the first week to let us know how things were going. The time seemed to drag and eventually Shirley spoke to her mum, but Kath sensed that there was something wrong. Mother's instinct, call it what you will, but when they returned it transpired they had run out of steroids the second week and Shirley had virtually spent the rest of honeymoon in her hotel room.

She looked really poorly when she got home and had a blinding headache so after a bit of a struggle we managed to put her to bed. David told us that Shirley had to be stretchered back onto the plane for the return journey home, because she was so ill. Shirley herself admitted, after recovering, that I had been right to tell them to book for just one week and that the heat in their room was almost unbearable, thus aggravating her itch.

With Dr Leonard's consent Shirley's daily drug intake and steroids were increased, and within a couple of days we saw a tremendous difference, with the lumps and bumps reduced. But her rally round was short-lived and Shirley began going downhill again, with the disease affecting her remaining lung quite badly. We were advised to keep an oxygen cylinder handy at all times, in case she became short of breath.

On one of her bad days in September 1995, I walked into Shirley's room and found her lying there with the oxygen mask, struggling for air, her eyes closed. When I sat on the end of the bed, she looked up at me and said it must be very difficult for us as her parents to see her in such distress.

Later that day I read The Sunday Mail and noticed they were asking for nominations for their annual "Great Scot" award for unsung heroes—people who had shown great courage or inspired others in a similar position. If there was ever a candidate for such an award, I thought, there was one right here: a real trooper who, despite all her trials, never moaned or complained. With this thought in mind I put pen to paper and nominated Shirley—without her knowing.

A few days later, I received a letter from Archie Mackay, the Sunday Mail's special projects editor, who asked for more information. I explained to him on the phone I would send photos of Shirley and David, as well as a copy of their wedding video. A couple of weeks later, Archie rang to say the newspaper were very interested in the nomination, but thought it would be better if Shirley knew what I was up to.

When I told her what I had done, she was horrified at the thought of a national newspaper being interested in her story, but after explaining my motives she understood. I was so proud of her and her attitude to others, and sharing her experience would encourage anyone in a similar position to take heart and fight with everything they had—just as she had done. I told Shirley her story would give people courage and inspiration, and perhaps lift them up from doom and gloom.

After consulting with David and her Mum, she agreed, if a little reluctantly, providing she was well enough at the required time. A couple of days later Archie came down from Glasgow and was completely overwhelmed by Shirley's honesty, both about her health and her future with David, neither of which looked very rosy.

All the nominees were to be judged by a prestigious panel and filmed just in case they were successful. Shirley was mortified when she found out that Scottish Television were coming down to film her and the family—especially because she had to wear a wig. Because it upset her so much, I called off the film session, explaining that she was too ill to appear in front of the camera.

However, after thinking it all over for a few days, Shirley said that if I thought she could help someone else, she would try and make the effort. The film crew arrived, along with the Sunday Mail's photographer, so the job could be done in a single day. Shirley literally had to drag herself from her sick bed that day, but was so determined to see things through.

Before her nomination could be submitted, she had to write her own account of how she felt. These are her words:

I'm not sure where to start my story . . . but I can tell you that before I was ill, I was like any normal 22 year old girl, with dreams and ambitions. Most of all I had a life I loved—full of horses, responsibility and independence.

In one day that all changed: from mucking out and riding one Thursday morning to a life-changing visit to the Borders General Hospital in the afternoon. My future from then on was in total turmoil. I remember feeling so scared not knowing what was wrong with me but also, deep down, knowing it was something serious. I had an inner feeling that this was no ordinary illness, but I was not ready for what we were to discover months later.

Numerous operations followed, and I have had needles in nearly every part of my body at one time or another, conscious and unconscious. The first was to be one of the worst: the lumbar puncture was everything the doctors had warned me about. I had to curl up on a bed and not move while they stuck a needle into my spine. My mum was there and I cried openly for most of the operation. It left me with a headache for two or three days that NO painkillers would shift. I was not eating, I could not think, my head was so sore and nobody could do anything. This was just the start. Once discovering the "problem" was not in my head, although I had previously been suffering headaches, they moved to my chest.

The doctors decided to try and take a biopsy from here as a shaded area had shown up on the X-ray. I was conscious again and this experience was another not to be forgotten. I felt like I was sitting on the roof watching a 30cm needle being slowly inserted into my body. I could not believe I was actually watching this procedure, but I was. I had a local anaesthetic but it had to be topped up a few times to stop the pain. As if that was not bad enough, as they were operating, air got into my lungs and I could not breathe properly: I could only pant. My pulse was going so fast, the vein on my neck was jumping. I was in so much pain I could not even cry and when I saw Mum and Dad after being stretchered out, I just wanted to reach out to them, and for Mum and Dad to take me me away from all this. Their faces said it all.

As this attempt was unsuccessful it was decided I should go to the City Hospital and get knocked out completely, to enable them to go in to see what was really going on and try another biopsy. I was there three days and my family and I were still unaware of what was about to surface. After my op I was put into the recovery room for a couple of hours. This was the first time my parents had seen me with tubes going everywhere on my by now thin body and an oxygen mask on my little face. When I was allowed to see them, they came in individually and I openly cried with relief.

But this operation confirmed the doctors' suspicions and brought the news that would change our lives forever: I had cancer. This happens in movies, I thought, not to someone you know and definitely not to yourself. I can't imagine what it was like for my Mum and Dad being told their only daughter—once lively and with a future but now a gaunt, dependent figure on a hospital bed—had the unmentionable "C" word.

The man to whom I was sent for treatment was the top consultant at the Western General Hospital. Dr Robert Leonard was to become my second dad and I owe my life to him—with a little will power and determination of my own, and lots of love and family support.

I was told of the treatment and its side effects more or less straight away, stupidly thinking I was ready to be sick occasionally and that my hair would fall out. I could not have been more wrong.

Weekly chemotherapy meant I had tablets to take at home: at one point I was taking between 20 and 25 daily. These made me feel more nauseated than actually sick. We had bought baseball caps, fancy hats and scarves in preparation for my hair loss, but I was not prepared for my emotions and sometimes they were more difficult to cope with. I baffled the doctors with my sheer will power and managed to keep going, even though I was getting thinner day by day. One morning I woke up and my hair started coming out in big clumps. I had thought, or hoped, at the time that I might have been the exception and kept mine.

I began wearing scarves and tried to act the same, but none of my clothes looked right with a hat and I became depressed. I hated looking in the mirror and cried all the time. I felt ugly, thin, sick, totally lacking in energy and thought that people didn't understand what I was going through. I could not even say the word "wig" as it implied something really false, but the nurses kept telling me about others who had tried them and after several gloomy months in hiding, I decided to have a go.

My own hair had been long and fair, but I always wanted to be a blonde so I thought I'd experiment and go a shade lighter. I liked the way I looked, although it was a bit strange having a wig and I worried in case it fell off, blew off, or someone snatched it. I always worried that a long lost friend would pull my hair jokingly, but to this day it has not happened.

I had now been given a Hickman Line, a tube that goes into my neck, round my heart and out at the top of my chest. It has three separate lines attached to it for giving treatment and taking blood samples. As I was now only six-and-a-half stone, my veins had totally packed in and this alternative was a godsend—until it became infected and all hell broke lose. I had to be whisked into hospital and put on antibiotics, a.s.a.p.

By this time I was wearing my blonde wig with a hat on top and I had started socialising again. I would look at other people in the pub and think, here I am, trying to look normal with barely no hair, a wig and hat, and a Hickman Line which most of the time was tucked into my bra. I thought how easy everyone had it, and it broke my heart to see girls running their hands through their hair.

It still does. My dream is to have my own hair again, long, like it used to be—not the kind you take off and hang on a chair!

There were times when I was well, then—as quick as a flash

—I was back in hospital if I got an infection or something. Having lost such a lot of weight, my job, which was also my hobby—riding—had gone completely out the window. Then one day I watched a video which gave me just the inspiration I needed. "Champions" is the true story of Bob Champion, the famous jockey who had cancer and fought to ride the famous racehorse Aldaniti in the Grand National. I watched and cried at this film many times, and felt we were in similar situations: we both wanted to live to ride again.

Now is the time to mention my beloved horse James, whom I looked after for four years when he was hunting. When I returned to my job at the stables, my boss decided to have a baby so the riding school closed down, and all the horses had to go back to their respective owners. James' "mum and dad", Sir Michael and Lady Sal Strang Steel lived close by, so I could still see James whenever I was able.

It was coming up to the hunting season again—August to February, and the Strang Steels needed a groom for James and their other horses and ponies. I was offered this position, with a flat just above the stables. I was so pleased to be with the horses I knew and loved and could not have wished to work for a kinder family. Unfortunately, my illness had other ideas and I became too weak even to lead the horses to the the field, never mind the hard physical work of mucking out, cleaning tack, riding and general management of these animals.

I will never forget the feeling I got—and sometimes still get—when I saw someone doing my job, with the horses I loved. It was something I had wanted, more than anything, at the time. Gradually I went down to watch less and less, as I felt I was in the way, and jealous that I did not have the energy to ride. I could only look and cry deep inside.

Thankfully, Lady Strang Steel knew how much I loved James and made it perfectly clear from the start that I was to treat him as my own and ride him whenever I felt like it. It would take me ages to get him, and myself, ready as I was so weak, and much as I loved him, I sometimes had to force myself to go. But boy, when I did, I felt normal and in control, and every time I rode over the hills it made me realise why I was fighting this illness.

We have an annual ride here in June, the Selkirk Common Riding, and I have done it every year since I was ten. This is what I was aiming for in 1993, a time of intense chemo and pills at home, but I was determined to do this ride. I told a very worried Mum and Dad my intentions and they both thought I'd be too ill when the time came. But I shocked them: I felt sick the whole week leading up to the Friday and sneakily stopped taking my pills on the Thursday—not that one day off tablets made me feel any better, I just thought that it did. On the day, James did his duty and more. What I owe to this horse for keepng my spirits going is too much to mention: I only hope and pray he can spend his retirement days with me to love and look after him, as he has done for me on so many occasions. (God bless you James, I love you.)

It took me a long while to recover from this major event, but at least I had done one thing I really wanted to do during my treatment.

The chemotherapy continued into 1994. During one particular course I was given very strong drugs for weeks at a time and I felt awful—a feeling I can still remember. My Mum slept on a make-shift bed next to mine because I had to have someone with me 24 hours day. I was sick every few minutes and did not sleep for weeks.

Getting an infection at a time like this, when your defences are very low, is life threatening and on a couple of occasions I had been written off, but something within kept me going. I fought for my Mum and Dad, always. They never gave up, so there's no way I could. Mum and I have always been very close, especially when I was younger and had ponies, but even when I became a teenager and interested in boys, she was like a sister and best friend rolled into one.

Dad and I were different. When I was small we lived in the country and he took me everywhere. When my friends were wandering the streets in groups, having fun and the odd spot of trouble, I was at home with the animals, going in the tractor or on the motorbike with Dad, or even just sitting in the house quite peacefully. I blame my shyness and some of my lack of self-confidence on this. I think I perhaps spent too much time on my own. Apart from that I would not change my childhood for anything.

We often laugh at the times I was carried out of hospital and laid on the back seat of the car, feeling rotten but wanting so much to come home, even for a few days. I love my family very much and would never have come through it all without this love, and our sheer determination that there is no way I can be taken away from them.

There has been more chemo and after the last session I was completely bald—a sight, especially if you are a girl and hair is your crowning glory. I hope none of you ever suffer this. Once, seeing myself this way, I felt distinctly inhuman—certainly not female anyway. Although I could put my hat on during the day and look relatively normal, you try standing in front of a mirror at night taking things off one by one: it's sheer hell. I felt like an alien that no-one could possibly love, or look at without being sick. Mum only saw this sight a couple of times and her reaction of tears, pity and sheer helplessness was enough for both of us. I spared my Dad this in case he would not be able to look at me—that would be even worse.

I've lost my hair four times now and it is currently the longest it has been for nearly three years. It's not long enough to go without a hat, but I'm hoping it will keep growing now and I'll get the hair I've always wanted.

Being ill is a lonely time, even if you have close famly and friends, but I have another pet to add to my "inspiration" list: my four-year-old cross breed dog, Skip. He came with me every day to the horses when I was working and never left my side at any other time. He comes in the car and I just hate leaving him when I go out because he looks so hurt. These days, because I am housebound energy-wise, he lies in our room, sleeping or just staring at me. I wonder what he thinks when I am crying: I'm sure he'd speak if he could. I don't think we give our animals enough credit for their intelligence and I believe they know more than we think.

In hospital, during a nasty bout of illness, I had an out-of-body experience when I went to heaven and came back. I was having some heavy duty chemo and decided that if this was life, then I'd be better off not being here. I had sometimes had thoughts about giving up but never seriously: now I was serious. I had to accept that with the treatment they could only try to keep me as well and pain-free as possible. I was on my own at the time, begging and praying to God and anyone else who might be listening. I was extremely sick and crying and remember saying I wanted to die.

Suddenly I had the weirdest feeling, but I also felt warm and safe. There were no "pearly gates" and someone waiting for me with open arms: I was in a place full of friendly people, crowding round and making me feel very welcome. Then I saw my Granny. She took me into her house and I was so happy there I did not want to come home.

When I was back in my bed, I remember feeling a great weight had been lifted and I knew that when my time came I was not going to be afraid—and I'm still not. I was unsure whether to write this as I know people will be sceptical. But it happened and I want people to know about it.

Now I just keep fighting with all I've got. I'd never have believed I could come this far through determination and sheer willpower, as at the start, I—and my Mum and Dad—did not think I'd be able to cope. Sometimes it's the shy people, who would not say "boo" to a goose, that have it inside when they need it. I can prove that.

People are so nice—well, my friends, anyway—even new friends who sympathise with our situation and get pleasure out of just being able to do something for us, however small. There are too many to mention but I owe immense thanks to each and every one. They don't realise how close I've felt to giving up when the phone rings and someone says: "Do you fancy riding my horse sometime?" Words to live for.

The last year has been the best and the worst for me. I have not had any ops for a while but my breathing is getting worse—bad enough to have an oxygen bottle and mask at my bedside. Even on good days I never get away from it as my medication is a surefire reminder. I carry a bag everywhere with me, full of all the essentials: not lipstick, hairbrush and perfume, but painkillers, steroids, creams and—the most important—morphine. I have not used it for a long time now but remember only too well the days when I was in such pain, with my back especially and my legs. I did not use the spoon, I just put the bottle to my mouth to get enough to numb the pain.

In this situation, I can think of nothing but being sore, watching Mum and Dad going out of the room to cry and compose themselves again before coming back to see me roll about on the bed screaming for the doctor. He gives me an enormous injection of morphine that completely knocks me out. I've taken spoonfuls of this everywhere—one night at the pictures I felt the pain coming on and did not want to miss the film.

It was during these episodes of being well and unwell that I met, and later married, the man of my dreams. Feeling ill is bad enough, but having very little hair and being so thin doesn't exactly make you feel like model material, and certainly not someone an eligible young man would want to go out with. But, as they say, "love is blind"! This amazing young man saw through everything and fell in love with the girl underneath, the one I'd lost, *because all I could see was the outside, and I hated myself. I was so far down but just when things are unbearable you get a little reprieve—and here he was.*

David is younger than me and I initially saw this as a huge problem—if I could not handle what was happening to me, how could someone younger? I was so afraid to get involved with anyone, as I knew getting attached, with all the hassles I had, would be very emotional, and I didn't know if I could handle it. But young or not, this guy was a tonic! He made me laugh on good and bad days, and I even started taking a little pride in myself again. At first I thought he just felt sorry for me or had a crush on an "older woman". I was wrong—he had fallen deeply in love.

We were friends for months and months and at first I could not imagine anything more serious because of our ages but I had to admit there was potential. I just had to be brave enough to trust him and hope that if it all fell through, I'd be OK.

He used to drive an old battered car around on two wheels (as young people do) but when he bought a smarter car, slowed down and changed out of his scruffy clothes, I thought it must be love!

Things were finally clinched when I was taken into hospital again and he travelled to Edinburgh every day, never leaving my side. He also helped Mum and Dad enormously at this time. Inevitably, our relationship strengthened and we were together every available minute. Soon age meant nothing and I too fell in love.

I rode the Marches at the Common Riding again this year and he stood with Mum and Dad, crying, as I rode in at the end with a huge smile on my face. I had been fine but then I started to cry too. I was proud of myself that day, something I've never admitted, and to tell the truth I think the people of Selkirk were rooting for me too.

There's no doubt that the treatment for cancer is terrible, but at least if you feel sick you can take a pill. If you're sore you can take painkillers, but if you're hurting emotionally you've had it. Nothing helps, because you are battling against yourself. Even now, I'll say I can handle the treatment, but not the side effects. I've seen psychologists, hypnotherapists and even a medium who sends me presents she thinks will help.

I am my worst enemy—I feel useless a lot of the time, because I can't work and probably never will again. I feel ugly because I don't have my own hair. Steroids give you more energy but they make you fat and the word "chipmunk" springs to mind.

Things looked very bleak for me healthwise for a few months and I had to face thinking about things I'd really like to do before I died. One was the Common Riding, which I accomplished. The second—far bigger and best ever—was my wedding day. Ever since I was a little girl I wanted to walk down the aisle on my Dad's arm and take my vows. This I managed to do in the space of just two months, with the help and dedication of Mum, Dad and numerous others. From white Rolls Royces to being piped into the church with my Dad, the day was fantastic and I have never been happier. The atmosphere was electric and everyone made the most of our special day.

It's now July 1995 and I've rallied round again from having breathing problems. It appears the doctors and tests say one thing, but each time my body has news for them. I have not been beaten yet and plan to keep fighting forever.

However, I admit to having more problems now than I had before. Because I love my husband very much and rely on him, I also fight for him, and if anything happened between us I know I'd want to give up. He has proved himself to me on countless occasions and I know he finds it so frustrating and hurtful when I tell him I don't trust him. I am afraid he will find someone better or just realise one day he's had enough of my illness, my moods, the crying and insecurity because when I am down I feel like I have the world on my shoulders. We must have a very strong love for each other but all I want in life is to be able to go out socially with him and for us to be so proud of, and at ease with each other, without having to worry in case an attractive girl comes in. Naturally, everyone turns to look at her—but I end up feeling ugly, horrible, boring and spoiling the night for us.

I just want to make David happy all the time. I'm always buying him pressies when he's at work to let him know I'm thinking of him while I am stuck at home, or if we've fallen out over something silly and I've been unreasonable. It's a good job we can stand back and look at the situation for what it is and that it's my illness that's causing it.

To sum him up, he's a gift from God: he's handsome, he oversees everything and loves me for me, not who I think or want to be or look like. He's part of me now, he's given me a life I'd lost way back and I want him to know just how special and important he is.

David, I love you and always will—I'll keep fighting for us, and our house in the country with stables and a garage for my Golf GTI, which I will definitely have one day!

Shirley A. Lowthian

The following week the Sunday Mail carried a double page spread about Shirley, calling her: "A Bride of Courage". Kath and I felt so humble and proud after reading the article, which underlined my belief that she would be an inspiration to any reader. A week later the editor of our local newspaper received the following letter . . .

"It is not with dry eyes I write this letter to you. The story of Shirley Lowthian is heartbreaking. How difficult it must be for her husband and parents, to reach out to such a beautiful wife and daughter, but we are powerless to change the way things are.

"I understand that no words of comfort can help Shirley or her family at this particular time, but my heart is with them, and like Shirley's Dad, I do believe in miracles. They say the Lord works in mysterious ways,

*and he only takes the good ones, so from what I have read
in the newspaper, he wants another little angel. To have
the courage and inner strength this family must have,
leaves the rest of us far behind.*

*"I will pray Shirley makes it for her award, if she is
lucky enough to win one, and we in the community will be
with her all the way. To me the greatest award given is life
itself, so why the threat of losing it to one so young, and
with so much to live for, is beyond all reason.*

*"I think I can safely say from the whole community
of Selkirk and beyond, to Shirley, David, Kath and Jim,
our heart and prayers go out to you, and you are always
in our thoughts.*

"Yours, (signed) A Heartbroken Parent."

Two weeks later, Archie from the Sunday Mail rang to tell us that
Shirley had made it to the last 12 finalists. This news in itself was
some achievement. She had been experiencing some really good and
really bad days again, and when Archie told us we had been invited
up to the awards dinner in Glasgow, irrespective of whether she had
won anything, we warned him how ill she really was. But Archie,
forever the optimist, said she would probably be OK on the night.
Shirley made the decision there and then that if she was unable to go
herself, she wanted her Mum and Dad to represent her and David.

In the week leading up to the dinner, however, none of us
intended to go because Shirley was so poorly. When we told Archie,
he pleaded with us to go and represent her. Towards the weekend,
Shirley said we must go, so we decided to organise a Macmillan
Nurse because she had never been left on her own before. Although
David would be there and was extremely capable, we wanted a nurse
on hand Just in case help was needed.

Before we set off for Glasgow, I promised Shirley that if her
story even got a mention, I would buy her the car of her dreams: a
Golf GTI. Where the money would come from I had no idea, but a
promise is a promise. We were accompanied that weekend by our
friends, Dennis and Hilda Murray, who had been very supportive

when things looked pretty grim. Shirley had also struck up a close relationship with them because they were outwith the immediate family and therefore she could confide in them.

When we arrived at the awards ceremony, after some pre—dinner drinks, the room was full of celebrity guests, including Ally McCoist, the Lord Provost of Glasgow, Lord McClusky, Lindsay Macdonald, Rory Bremner and Gavin Hastings, to name but a few. The four of us felt that had Shirley been able to attend, she would have taken the place by storm.

The atmosphere from the start was electric and it was very emotional, listening to all the stories of raw courage, and how people had confronted adversity. When the film about Shirley was shown, it was just too much for me and I was not afraid to shed a tear—even in front of the 600 people in the audience—for my daughter, who was very sick back home in Selkirk. The film received rapturous applause, and it was then revealed that Shirley had indeed won an award, which would be presented by Gavin Hastings, then captain of the Scotland rugby squad.

I had never spoken to an audience before—except at the wedding—but promised I would read out a small speech which Shirley had prepared if she was lucky enough to win something . . .

> *"It would have been an honour to have been here tonight. Unfortunately, I am not well enough, but firstly I would like to thank Dr Leonard, my consultant, and the staff at the Western General Hospital in Edinburgh for keeping me going—especially Dr Leonard, who is like a second father to me. I often have to ask his permission to go places and do things.*
> *"But mostly I want to thank my Mum and Dad and my new husband David, because if it were not for their love, support and determination, I might not be still here. Thank you."*

I really struggled to finish the speech, as I held the lovely engraved Caithness crystal trophy in the shape of a thistle, but managed to add a few words of my own . . .

> *"Shirley has managed to get her message across to anyone ill that all is not doom and gloom. Yes, it is a shock to the system, but she is living proof that where there's life, there's hope, especially in 1995, where great advances are being made in the fight against cancer.*
>
> *"Last but not least, a special mention must go to Shirley's Mum, who gave the special nursing care and attention only a Mum can give. I do not think Shirley or I could have made it through the last few years without her."*

The ceremony was handled in a very sensitive way and people were very kind to us that night, stopping us in the hall and sending their love and best wishes to Shirley and David.

We managed to phone Shirley after the presentations and she was absolutely thrilled when we told her she had won an award. When we eventually said goodnight, she promptly reminded me about the car, and I told her we would speak about it the next day.

It was 3am when Kath and I went to bed, but I was woken at 6am by Kath sobbing. She was standing at the hotel window, clutching the trophy, and said she wished she was back home with Shirley. We arrived home at lunchtime on the Sunday, to be greeted by a delighted Shirley and David. Although we had only been away overnight, it seemed like a lifetime.

Chapter Four:

A TEST OF FAITH

O ur little lass was letting me know in no uncertain terms that she was determined to have her beloved car, as she had sent David to the local Volkswagen dealer to pick up a brochure on Golf GTIs. As ill as she was, the excitement at the prospect of them getting the car of their dreams was electric. When I think back it was one of the best decisions Kath and I made, because they really needed cheering them up.

The planned extension to the house was put on the back burner, but we knew where our priorities lay. After getting the necessary bank loan, the hunt was now on for the car, which had to be green or black, Shirley's favourite colours, and have the Golf GTI badge on the grille.

Shirley was having trouble now with blood clotting in her leg. One day it was so swollen, it was nearly twice the size of the other leg. I called Dr Leonard and he immediately insisted on seeing her the following day, resulting in Shirley being put on anti-clotting agents. She had to be kept in hospital so the agents could be given to her slowly, intravenously.

Severe headaches, numbness to her face and some loss of hearing also beset Shirley at this time. She had to take various drugs to combat the symptoms, caused by the glands in her neck being so swollen that they affected the nerves in the side of her face. This further produced problems in one of her eyes, making it impossible for her to watch TV or read. I came up with the idea of taking one lens out of a pair of dark sunglasses, and placing cotton wool over the other side. It helped a little, but in all honesty it broke our hearts to see her wearing them.

We were now coming up against things we had not encountered before. Shirley's sore heads became so painful she could not lift her head off the pillow: she was even afraid to move. Her teeth were also affected and she had constant toothache.

A scan was called for to see what was happening in her head and neck but a waiting list meant a delay of three weeks, and more pain and suffering for Shirley. The brochure of her car was pinned above her bed, and when things were really bleak she would glance up at the picture, and give a wry kind of smile.

When the time came for the scan, Shirley was so ill she could not travel in the car up to Edinburgh, so an ambulance was called. However, she was able to make the return journey by car and told us she was worried about the latest test results.

Because she thought she was ugly compared to other women, Shirley was crying quite a lot now. We tried to reassure her but it was difficult, even when her own hair had grown back in, as it wasn't the same glossy hair as in the days before her illness.

I was always the last to go to bed as my final task of the day was to walk the dogs. When I passed Shirley and David's door on the way upstairs, I always said, "Goodnight, guys". The reply would come back: "Goodnight, Jim," followed by: "'Night, Dad". I got a lot from that. Like Kath, I would cry upstairs in the privacy of our room—our thoughts were always with the "kids" below.

Two days later we received a dreadful blow: the scan showed the disease was now on Shirley's brain and behind her nose, causing the numbness in her face. Radiotherapy would be tried next but it was difficult because it would be near so many vital organs.

As Christmas was fast approaching, I telephoned my friend Joe at his garage in Glasgow to see if he had been able to find a suitable vehicle. Happily he had tracked down one on the other side of the city. Our idea was to keep it a secret and pretend we could not find a car in time for Christmas, but Shirley was feeling so low that we decided to tell her.

We found the following entry in her diary later:

THURSDAY 2:32 pm (just before Christmas)—Xmas is just four days away and is perfect in nearly every way. I'm with my family, who I love, and the first Xmas with my husband. It's snowing, and I'm getting the car of my dreams. I only wish I was well. God, please let me be well enough over Xmas for everyone to enjoy themselves, and let me be in not too much pain. That's the most important Xmas present I want. PLEASE HELP. I'll fight if you give me a hand every now and again, God. SHIRLEY XXXX

We travelled up to Edinburgh every day for treatment, which meant going to two different departments, one for a strong dose, the other for a weak one. Shirley instructed us to watch closely after she came out of the first treatment, because she had noticed that it caused her toenails and fingernails to turn blue.

She was now wheelchair bound, weak and very thin, and one day I had to turn back because she felt so unwell. The daily journey was tough on her, even though the treatment lasted only a few minutes. Once more, the radiotherapy meant Shirley would lose all her precious hair.

I was now literally having to carry Shirley to and from the car. Her headaches were quite bad now and when we got home she only wanted to go into a darkened room, to get some relief.

A couple of days before Christmas I caught her in tears in her room and when I asked her what was wrong, she said it was the first time in her illness she had not been able to go and buy Christmas presents herself. As usual Mum managed to work something out, with both of us doing some shopping on Shirley's behalf.

It was snowing quite hard on Christmas Eve, the day the car arrived. It was a cracker, but we decided to hide it in a friend's garage just around the corner. Kath and I planned to put a big ribbon round it, with a card, and some messages on the windows. As we got to work on the car, we just glanced at each other, knowing Shirley might not ever be well enough to drive it. The insurance would come into effect on January 19th, her 25th birthday.

On Christmas morning, we took the youngsters some breakfast and exchanged some presents, but Shirley was unwell, and we knew she would have to make a special effort if she was going to enjoy the day. Soon that twinkle appeared and she looked at us, as if to say: where is my car, then, folks?

We told her to wait a few minutes and we would get it for her. We arrived back at the front door to find her fully dressed, with David on her arm and a great big smile on her face. It was wonderful to see something that had been missing for such a long time.

The car was a "K" registration and I don't think Shirley had expected to get one quite so new. Kath led her by the hand to the car for a seat while I snapped away with the camera. We crossed the road to get a better view of her sitting in the car, but noticed she had her hands crossed on the steering wheel, and her head on her hands, crying her eyes out. She said she was so happy and had everything she could ever want, except her health. If money could have bought it for her, we would have sold everything we had.

Barring a miracle, we knew we would not spend another Christmas together. We sat round the table for dinner, and even although we tried our best, we all felt a bit glum. Despite Shirley's extra effort, she felt unwell and had to go back to bed. It was difficult because her itchy legs and feet, a symptom of the disease, were driving her crazy. We knew her tears were borne out of frustration rather than complaints.

The final week of Shirley's treatment just after Christmas was to be spent in hospital, as she was too weak to travel. David stayed with her throughout, and we went up every day. The enforced stay brought some dividends, however, because she was given treatment for her sore heads, and there was a slight improvement in her hearing. Midway through January, Shirley's eyesight also got better, so we all felt as though we were on the up.

However, the optimism was short-lived. Shirley was put back onto chemo, as her breathing was becoming quite difficult, and she began taking quite a lot of oxygen again. A pain in her ribcage appeared, so Mum strapped it up, thinking she had maybe popped a rib with all her violent coughing. But this didn't ease matters much and Shirley soon had to go back on quite a high dose of morphine to lessen the pain, and calm her a little to settle her lungs. With antibiotics on the scene now as well, things were looking a bit bleak again.

The night after Shirley's 25th birthday she got dressed and asked me to take her for a drive in her new car, to Galashiels and back. En route she became so ill we had to turn back. She later managed a quick drive to Sir Walter Scott's favourite scenery, Scott's View, but I think that was about the only time she drove her beloved car.

Early February saw her health deteriorate, with more antiobiotics, oxygen, morphine and regular blood checks. Depression set in with a vengeance, and her doctor tried antidepressants to see if that would help. Shirley was now crying quite a lot, with an intensity we had never encountered during her entire illness.

The pressure was getting to David as well, but if I told you what that young lad had endured during his wife's bouts of depression, you would probably run a mile. It wasn't our daughter's character and David knew it, so he stuck by Shirley through thick and thin. Kath and I just stood by and admired him, and often told him so.

Fight as Shirley did, she was now completely bedridden, and breathlessness was forcing her to use the oxygen bottle. There was nothing Kath and I could do except be there for her. Our faith was really being tested now.

Our lass was now so ill that appointments with Dr Leonard were being missed, which drove her even deeper into depression, as he had always managed to say the right things and perk her up a little.

Her close friends stood by her in these dreadful times, although sometimes Shirley did not want to see anyone. They respected her wishes, and were content just to sit in the next room, although after their visits, we always told her who had popped in.

The strain on the three of us was immense at this point. I began to think we were entering the final stages of this nightmare, with this horrible disease finally claiming our girl. We had never been through a period like this; it was a time in which Shirley could not face any more treatment and hope appeared so distant. She would only take morphine or sleeping pills, to sleep her days away.

These hours spent at rest during the day revived Shirley and she seemed to come alive during the evenings for a while. She even attempted to eat something—but she only managed negligible amounts. David was spending all night making sure she had oxygen as and when she needed it.

To cheer her up, I had written to the SRU, to try and obtain tickets for the Grand Slam decider between Scotland and England at Murrayfield. Kath and I new she would never make it, but nevertheless we received two tickets for the match, and a kind letter from Duncan Paterson, the then Chief Executive and his wife Lucille. I also organised for Shirley to meet Noel Edmonds after his show in Ayr but again she was too ill to go.

Only parents in Kath and I's position could ever possibly know the pain and anguish we were going through at this particular time. A piece of us—and David—was literally dying in the bedroom next door every day and I cannot describe just how I felt then.

Sal Strang Steel must have heard how ill Shirley was, because she came to see her and said that her beloved James was waiting for her to take him round the Common Riding again that year. If she could not come and see him, Sally would bring him down to her window.

Call it instinct, intuition or whatever, but on the 2nd April, 1996, none of us attempted to go to work, not even for ten minutes, because suddenly Shirley became desperately ill and was virtually gasping for air. By chance her doctor called for an impromptu visit and examined her for what seemed like ages. He beckoned for the three of us to go into the kitchen and explained that the last good piece of Shirley's lung was severely infected and she would probably take bronchial pneumonia, which would ultimately lead to her death. He wanted to take her into hospital, but we expressed her wish that when the time came, she wanted to be at home with us. Reluctantly he agreed to her request, but insisted that he increase her morphine, perhaps even with a touch of heroin, to try and stop her gasping for breath.

When the doctor left, the three of us stood in the kitchen for a few minutes, crying and cuddling each other. It was the most terrible news and I was overwhelmed with compassion for my wife Kath—all those years she had so tenderly taken care of our beautiful child, while I was at work. Now God had decided to take her from us, and there was nothing we as a family could do to prevent it.

We knew now that we had to be really strong for Shirley, as there were tough and unthinkable times ahead. When I returned to her room, I looked at her with the oxygen mask on, gasping for air and had to leave momentarily, as I choked back the tears.

One of the first jobs the doctor had given me was to make sure Shirley had a plentiful supply of oxygen 24 hours a day. Going into her room and hearing the oxygen hissing is a sound I will never forget.

Shirley was now discussing the future with David. He was only a young man, she said, and she thought he should leave Selkirk and join the forces after she died, as he had always wanted to be a mechanic. She also told him he would probably have other relationships, but David said whatever the future held, he would never love anyone else the way he loved her.

The local district nurse was now coming in daily to change Shirley's drugs in the pump attached to her arm. We took turns sitting up at night with her, while David slept upstairs, afraid he would turn round in the middle of the night and disconnect the intravenous pump by mistake. He was also troubled when she started coughing because now it was certain to turn into a coughing fit, which was even very scary to Kath and I.

Shirley seemed to get a lot of comfort lying on her side facing the wall, because often when entering her room, I would say: "You all right, Shirl?" Then a hand would appear from under the covers, and give a cheeky wave.

She wanted to spend time alone that week, and we now know that she was sorting a lot out in her head. One night she asked to see Hilda and Dennis Murray, as they were in the house. Dennis went through hesitantly, not wanting to disturb Shirley, but was surprised to see her sitting up in bed, "holding court"—not the sickly person he had expected.

During this time Shirley appeared to come to terms with her condition, and as she had prepared herself, she was now preparing us. On April 5th she was so brave, actually choosing her favourite green as the colour of her coffin lining. She also wanted to be buried in her Mum's tartan nightdress with her wedding rings on, and some of her favourite cuddly toys beside her.

Shirley went on to pick the cord bearers and apart from David and myself, we knew there would be a few surprised faces at the other choices—her blacksmith, Charles Smith Maxwell (husband of her former boss Sandra), Sir Michael Strang Steel, and David's eldest brother Iain. Keith Williamson, Shirley's first real love from her teenage years, was also to be present at the graveside. We knew a few eyebrows would be raised but it didn't matter what people thought because our lass was so brave to even think about what lay ahead.

It was Saturday night, April 6th, and I was with her when she tried to get to her comfy position facing the wall. I noticed her spine as she was turning and it was so thin it would have made the strongest man cry. I knew she was changing by the hour, and it was not for the better.

As her immediate family, we were praying to anyone who would listen. You feel so alone at times like these and when you glance out the window you seem to notice that everyone and everything goes on as before, as though your problems do not exist.

I had been working on the gates to my business premises, close to my house, when the nurse who was making her daily call on Shirley, stopped for a chat. With hindsight, the subject was about loss, something that hitherto had not even entered my head. Even though my daughter was so ill, I could not comprehend losing her, and was clinging desperately to the idea that something would turn up at the last minute.

All we could give Shirley was her favourite drink, Ribena. Earlier in her illness, when she had been unable to eat, it appeared to sustain her but it was not enough now.

Shirley was now so ill it was heartbreaking to even enter her room. On Sunday, April 7th, we had to call out the doctor as she was having severe nose bleeds, but we did not know if it was coming from her nose or elsewhere in her body.

The nurse came in later that day, and when we told her Shirley was taking liquid morphine to try to sleep, she called the doctor for permission to increase the dosage in the pump on her arm.

Kath and I felt like crying every time we looked at her in her room. That evening, we chased David upstairs to bed because he was exhausted, worried and needed a bloody good cry. Kath was lying under the duvet with Shirley; I was sprawled out on a chair, feet on the edge of the bed, and at 1a.m. Shirley appeared to be in a talkative mood, asking us the name of the actor in A Few Good Men, among other trivia. Kath gave up at about 3 am and went to bed as well, but not before telling Shirley she was a "wee blether". Shirley said she would be OK because I was with her.

The early hours on Monday, April 8th, were spent with me passing cotton wool to wipe the blood from Shirley's face as her nose would not stop bleeding. All through this dreadful episode she never complained or moaned, although she had every reason to do so. It was the longest night I have ever spent, and the sheer feeling of helplessness was terrible, because all I could do was be there.

When I saw Kath at 7:30 am, I told her I thought we needed professional help now, because I felt I could not handle the previous night's experience again, as it was breaking my heart to see Shirley in so much distress. I was now beginning to lose it, and wasn't afraid to admit it.

After his call that morning, the doctor said he was worried about Shirley as her platelets were so low, and as there was a distinct possibility she could haemorrhage, he wanted her to go into hospital. Once more we had to be brave and express Shirley's wishes. Her courage knew no bounds, because we put his suggestion to her, and she firmly said: "No".

After the drug in her arm was increased once more, Shirley turned to her mum and said: "Don't worry mum, everything will be all right and I will die tonight." We knew we could not let her down when she needed us most, so we dug deep into our resources.

It was now unbearable to watch Shirley lying helplessly in bed, trying to take a drink of water. She squeezed my hand on one occasion, more or less to say, don't worry Dad. Shirley asked her mum, "Is it OK if I go today Mum?" and she said, "it's OK, Shirl, we'll be with you to the end".

Kath and I left her for a couple of minutes to have a cup of tea next door, when a voice as clear as day said, "Mum". We dashed into the room and Kath sat on the bed, embracing Shirley in her arms. She asked her if she wanted a drink, but our poor Shirley turned her head ever so slightly and said, "No, Mum, it's the other". Kath replied, "Do you just want a cuddle?" Shirley said, "Yes Mum", and died in her mother's arms. The arms that held her as she came into this world were holding her as she left.

I was holding on to Shirley's feet at the bottom of the bed when she died, just wanting to be near her and touch her. The district nurse called and checked Shirley, confirming that she had died and left us on our own in the room while she called the doctor.

Kath and I just cried uncontrollably with heartache, frustration, grief and relief for poor Shirley. It was a living nightmare.

One of the hardest phonecalls I ever had to make was to David, who had popped out to his mum's for a message. On arriving home the young lad was absolutely devastated.

As grief stricken as Kath was, she insisted on preparing Shirley for the arrival of the undertaker herself, a task only a devoted mother could do.

Even though we were all going about in a daze, there was much to do. There was the difficult task of informing the family, because even finding the words to say that Shirley had died was dreadful. I could hardly string two words together when I told my business partner's wife, and that day the branches of our business were closed as a mark of respect. My partner Robert Smyly called to see me on his way back from work and offered all the assistance I needed. At a time like that true friends really show their mettle.

On Tuesday, David and I went to make the arrangements at the registrar's—with the same lady that had helped arrange Shirley and David's wedding banns. She was visibly shocked when told of

Shirley's death and halfway through the paper work began sobbing, losing her professional composure for a few moments.

We both met people in the street that day—they just came up to us looking stunned. All said they were thinking about us and expressed their sorrow that Shirley lost her life after such a brave fight.

When I went to the undertakers that night to see Shirley for the last time, I cannot explain how I felt as her father, seeing her so peaceful, so at rest, with all the pain and stress gone. The lump in my throat was so large I could hardly breathe. I kissed her on the forehead, and held her little hand, as I said my last farewells. My faith was now being tested to the limit, but I really did believe Shirley was in heaven with God, and to this day I still believe that.

The next day the Sunday Mail asked if they could come down to do a special tribute to Shirley. The only reason we agreed was because she would have wanted it, in case it would help some other poor soul in a similar predicament.

The days leading up to the funeral were harrowing and many tears were shed. There were so many pictures of Shirley on the wall, not just because she was ill but because her Mum loved photos and they all served as a poignant reminder of the daughter we had lost.

The night before her burial, Shirley came home. I had warned Kath and David that it would be pretty upsetting, but they were just so pleased that she was back with us, even if it was only for a while. Kath adorned the room with candles and Shirley looked so at peace, her faithful dog Skip sitting by her coffin.

I could not cope with the terrible grief I was feeling, and her loss was too much to take. I spent the night in Shirley's room with her, as I knew it would be for the last time, and just lay and thought about all the good times—and some of the bad times—we had had.

The day of the funeral dawned and when I saw Kath's family arrive outside the house, it was enough to start me off again. I pulled myself together and met them downstairs in an emotional reunion. How Kath held herself together God only knows—David as well. I had written some words but would be too distraught to speak at the funeral, so the minister, Rev. David Kellas, agreed to say them for me.

There was many more people than Kath and I had expected at the church. Many of Shirley and David's friends turned up to give her a good farewell. There weren't many dry eyes in the church, which was full.

Kath and I had chosen the hymns, "Abide With Me" and "All Things Bright and Beautiful". David had also asked his elder brother—a professional musician—to play the love song he had written for their wedding. When we heard it we just gave way to our emotions—it was such a beautiful and fitting tribute to two young people. The Minister gave a lovely service, as he had done at their wedding.

It was a sad and emotional day when we laid Shirley to rest, but the hundreds of beautiful cards and floral tributes showed how highly she had been regarded. It helped us through what was a difficult time.

Kath showed incredible courage—perhaps that's where our brave Shirley got her mettle. Not many mums and dads see their only daughter married, then bury her nine months later, leaving their son-in-law a widower at only 20 years of age.

The next day I felt absolutely gutted. I started crying and could not stop, until I reminded myself that Shirley was now free from all the pain and hurt. I think the realisation of this helped.

We kept visiting the cemetery—a natural response, I think—but the grief and emptiness I was feeling would not stop, especially when I was on my own. The enormity of it all began to sink in: we would not see Shirley again.

David went to London with his elder brother Iain for a few days, and Kath and I resolved to attempt to go into work at the end of that week.

The break-up of Shirley's flat was heart rending and terrible. Clearing it out made everything so final. As I was tidying up things in her room, I came upon a note she had placed between the pages of a book. It was her will. It read: "I do not have much, but this is what I would like to happen to those things I do own. If anything should happen to me, I want David, Mum and Dad to take what clothes they would like to keep, then give the rest to homeless charities. I would like my faithful dog Skip to stay with my parents, but would like David to come and take him out sometimes."

At the end of April, David moved his belongings out of the house. He looked really dejected and down. After he left, the room looked so terrible and empty, just like everything else in our lives at that moment.

We also had to call the blacksmith, Charlie Cockburn, out to Shirley's old ponies, Birchie and Wedding Bells, to pare their feet. Charlie went back a long way with Kath and Shirley, in fact all the way back to their early pony club days. He said afterwards that the two old ponies had probably come through their last winter. Birchie, now 29, would perhaps have to be put to sleep in November, along with his old companion who was now 32. It was a terrible thing for us to consider but they could not stand another winter.

When the time came we decided to dig a grave in the corner of their field, so they could be buried where they had grazed for the last seven years. The only thing that made it bearable was that Shirley would be reunited with her old friends once more.

Her dream car was sent back to Glasgow, because it was heartbreaking for us to see it sitting at the back of the house. I watched it go, and that night Kath and I had a bloody good cry.

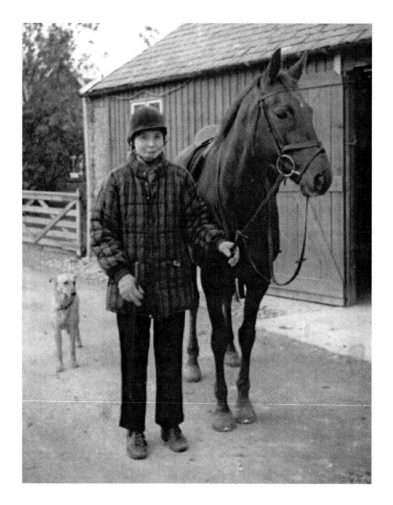

Shirley in the autumn of 1995, outside her old stables at Lindean.

Chapter Five:

LIFE WITHOUT SHIRLEY

The loss of Shirley soon began to really sink in. I kept thinking she had gone away and would walk in the door any day now. Kath and I hid a lot of our feelings from our friends, colleagues and family. We began to hate the weekends which simply provided too much time to dwell on things.

I watched a video, made the previous year, of Shirley working out on her beloved James and to see her talking, moving and riding was something to cherish. I thank God for whoever invented the camcorder.

Kath lost her composure in public for the first time when we went to the Gyle Shopping Centre near Edinburgh, a favourite of Shirley's, probably because Shirley had walked along the very same paths and stairways we were walking now. We left after 25 minutes or so.

We promised to be strong for Shirley but increasingly we felt that if this was life without our daughter, you can keep it, because everything was now meaningless and empty.

We truly struggled with the seemingly endless hours stretching ahead of us day after day. Eventually, in an effort to occupy all this time on our hands, Kath and I decided to start fund-raising for Shirley's favourite charity, the Scotland and Newcastle Lymphoma Group. It would at least give us some purpose in life and we would be doing something worthwhile.

Kath and I tried to focus our minds by arranging a fund-raising evening at the end of August. We were able to book the band who had played at Shirley's wedding, the Strangers, who generously waived their fee. Donations from the public also began to come in, which cheered us up a little. If Shirley had been with us, she would have been delighted.

To tell the truth, I felt—and often still feel—that if I did not have such events to work towards, life could be very difficult to face. Kath and I have spent many a miserable weekend when we have just longed for Monday to come round again.

From time to time, we got visits from people, such as Fiona, the nurse from the Western General Hospital, and Archie Mackay from the Sunday Mail. We appreciated these very much, but even such kind gestures of concern could not lift the terrible sadness and grief inside both Kath and I. On more than one occasion I have come home at lunch time to find Kath crying—her tears a release for a 'bad day'and the burden she now carries always.

My diary at that time reflects the unceasing anguish we were feeling: "I walk the dogs morning, noon and night, and I do everything to choke back the tears. But if I start crying during the day, I don't think I could cope with work. The next person that tells me life goes on will actually make me sick. I know they mean well, but unless they have been through such an ordeal themselves, they don't know what they are talking about. I tell them to imagine one of their children dying, and multiply that feeling 1,000 times. Then they just might have an inkling of how Kath, David and I feel."

June 3, 1996, was a very big day for us as we plucked up the courage to remove Shirley's bed from the house. It was heartrending, as this was the end of another chapter in our lives. We managed to get through it somehow, but unfortunately I now felt as if I was waiting for something: for Shirley to come back from holiday, or just to wake up and find that this was just one horrible nightmare.

Everyone in the town had started to ride their horses in preparation for the Common Riding on the 14th, and I just could not imagine it without our Shirley. The following weekend was one of the worst yet, as Kath and I were doing a lot of crying. We ordered a nice floral display for Shirley's grave, in the shape of a rosette, for the coming weekend.

We woke up at 4am on the Common Riding morning, to hear the bands going round the town to wake the Standard Bearer and Provost, as tradition demands. Kath, understandably, was quite upset when she left for work. Perhaps she felt she had to hide away because it was too distressing for her to be in Selkirk on Shirley's special day.

I went to the cemetery at 9:30 am and sat at the side of Shirley's grave, to watch for the horses to come over the hills. The empty feeling inside was as bad as the day she had died. I spoke to her in the hope she could perhaps hear me, and stayed with her until every horse had returned to the town. Silly old fool, some people might think, but I did not have the heart to leave her alone on her special day. Somehow we managed to get through that difficult weekend—I just wished there was an easy way of getting through them all.

Rather than easing as time went on, the pain of our loss appeared worse during that summer. Only a year previous we had been getting ready for her wedding . . . We both cried at nights in different rooms, quietly enough so that one couldn't hear the other. My secretary got married on July and we attended the ceremony, but all Kath and I could think of was Shirley's wedding. We kept thinking she has just gone off on holiday and any minute she will walk through the door and say, "mum, dad, I'm home".

In the early months of our bereavement, we were introduced to the local branch of a group known as The Compassionate Friends, which aims to support parents who have lost a child. It was heartrending when Kath and I went to our first meeting, as we saw the hurt and pain on the faces of people just like us. We had all set out to bring up our respective families, unaware that all our hopes and plans would come to nothing when each one of us had to face the ultimate nightmare for any parent—the death of a child.

Since those blackest of days, we have been moved by many acts of kindness, great and small. For example, Kirkhope Primary School at Ettrickbridge donated their Christmas collection, and in return, we offered to present the Shirley Lowthian Memorial Shield annually to the child who has worked the hardest or made a significant improvement to their work. Another regular event is the mixed charity bowls tournament at Ettrick Forest Bowling Club, which takes a great deal of organisation and hard work behind the scenes.

Yet another event was inspired by a chance encounter. In the summer of 1996 a young lad from Manchester noticed a collecting can on the counter of the Cross Keys bar in Selkirk, owned by our good friends Dennis and Hilda Murray. They told him who Shirley was and how she died, and on his return to Manchester, the young lad related the story to fellow members of his football team, the Vulcans. Even though they had never met Shirley, they were adamant they would make a contribution in some way, and arranged to play Selkirk Football Club during a three-day event in May 1997. It was planned that the Vulcans would arrive on the Friday, play football on the Saturday, enjoy an evening disco, and play golf on the Sunday. Happily, it was a great success and the Vulcans visited us again in 1998, raising £1600 through their efforts.

For the 1999 charity football weekend, the Selkirk club not only played host to the Vulcans but also a team from Holland and another from Lothian and Borders Police. On that occasion, the tournament was won by the home team and once again was a resounding success, paving the way for other similar events in the future.

Each October, a fund-raising dance is held at the Victoria Hall in Selkirk, with Shirley's favourite band The Strangers which ensures a large following. An auction and raffle are also held at the dance, where items such as rugby shirts donated by the Scottish team further boost the funds for the SNLG. At the time of going to print, almost £17,000 has been raised for the charity over the last three years.

While the fund-raising has provided a welcome focus for us and the results are tremendously rewarding, our loss is never far below the surface. It's just when you think things are getting a little better that your emotions sneak up on you, and coupled with grief, they are terrible to deal with. I often wonder how people would react if they knew that sometimes, when we were talking to them and looking calm on the outside, we were actually screaming inside with the pain and hurt at the loss of our beautiful daughter.

One day I plucked up enough courage to go and pick up some of Shirley's riding gear from the stables where she was given horses to ride during her illness. Just to touch her things brought memories flooding back.

We planned a holiday abroad in October, 1996, not knowing if it was for the best or not. I hate flying, but Kath and I told ourselves that if the plane dropped into the sea, we had nothing left to live for anyway.

We hoped that the first Christmas without Shirley would pass as quickly as possible. Even the thought of a Christmas card on the wall made us want to break down and cry. We decided not to buy any presents that year, and just prayed that people would understand.

Priorities in life have changed dramatically for us: everything generally held to be 'important'—possessions, money, social life, holidays—mean nothing at all when you have lost someone you love. People say we should move on, and we know that, but to actually do it is a different thing.

We have been comforted greatly in the knowledge that at each Selkirk Common Riding, Shirley's love of all things equestrian lives on through the annual bequeathing of a sum of money in her memory to be put towards the horse expenses of the Royal Burgh Standard Bearer. The Shirley Lowthian Memorial Fund will continue into the new millennium, ensuring that she will always be involved in her favourite time of the year—she will always be there in spirit.

The cutting edge of the fund-raising aspect—medical research—has also commanded my attention over the past three years. I follow, with interest, the progress reported in various charity bulletins and newsletters. In 1998 Kath and I gave the University of Edinburgh Medical School permission to ask questions about Shirley's past life, as they have been trying to find out why so many people catch Hodgkins' Disease. We hope our answers will help them in their efforts.

All these facets have helped Kath and I make sense of our lives over recent years—such focal points have been a lifeline, allowing us to collect our shattered thoughts and emotions and channel them purposefully. But throughout this time I have carried yet another—much greater and more personal—need which has continued to demand my attention. Ever since Shirley died I have been compelled to tell her story and I suppose the many hours I spent keeping a diary, and writing material for the book, provided an outlet for my emotions and helped me in the grieving process. I told Shirley I planned to write a book about her and I think she was a bit sceptical at the time, but if she thought it would help someone else in a similar situation, I know she would have supported me all the way.I confided in a few people who could perhaps help me get the book published, and once I had done this, I knew there was no going back. The project gathered momentum and soon took on a life of its own. I was determined to get it into print for Shirley's sake, and to help raise funds for the Scotland and Newcastle Lymphoma Group. Soon a publishing date was set for the end of 1999, three-and-a-half years after Shirley's death.

At the time of going to print, my emotions are on a different level. We still find it hard to accept we will never see our beloved daughter again, and find special events like Christmas, birthdays and holidays especially difficult. Sometimes we just go about in a daze, living in what you might call a robotic fashion. Without our charity work I think things would be even worse. I often look at

Kath and try to imagine the hurt and unbearable sense of loss she must be feeling each and every day.

We often told Shirley when we went into her room that people were sending her their love. She told us that if love was a cure in itself, she was being sent enough to cure everyone in both the Western and Borders General Hospitals put together.

Sadly, love was not enough and although Shirley won many a battle during her illness, I'm afraid the war was just too much. That's not to say that the outlook is bleak for everyone with Hodgkins' Disease, because at this very moment, excellent medical teams at both the Western and the BGH are working hard to help people beat this illness, and there are many success stories to tell.

God must have had a reason for taking Shirley from us, but in her final days she assured us she was not frightened of the journey which lay ahead, as she would be waiting for us all to be together again one day.

Kath, David and I, and all her friends and family, will miss her dearly and so will everyone else who was ever touched by her vivaciousness and zest for life.

Although this book has focussed mainly on Shirley's illness, I know she would like to be remembered as the bubbly young blond charging about on her pony over the hills of Lindean, with her favourite collie dog running after her. We remember her this way, but we cannot forget the difficult years during which she fought her illness with such bravery. This book is a lasting testament to Shirley's courage, and now, the greatest reward for us would be that someone who is fighting a similar battle will be inspired by her story.

I'm Free

Don't grieve for me, for now I'm free
I'm following paths God made for me
I took his hand, I heard him call
Then turned, and bid farewell to all.

I could not stay another day
To laugh, to love, to sing, to play
Tasks left undone must stay that way
I found my peace . . . at close of day.

And if my parting left a void
Then fill it with remembered joy
A friendship shared, a laugh, a kiss
Ah yes, these things I too will miss.

Be not burdened . . . deep with sorrow
I wish you sunshine of tomorrow
My life's been full . . . I've savoured much
Good friends, good times, a loved one's touch.

Perhaps my time seemed all too brief
Don't lengthen it now with undue grief
Lift up your heart and share with me
God wants me now . . . He set me free.

Author Unknown

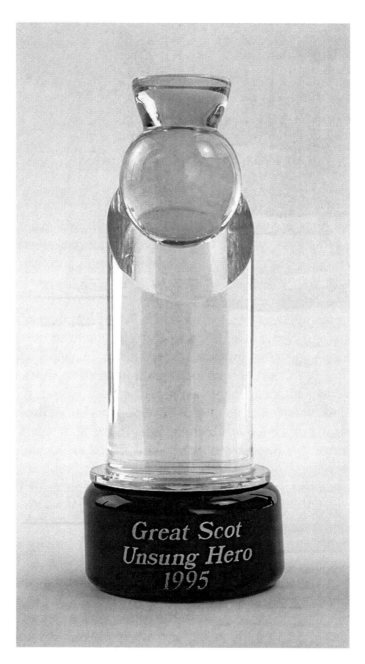

Photo: Penny Davies Photography

Appendix:

LYMPHOMA: The Facts

L ymphomas are cancers of the lymphoid cells, which are part of the lymphatic system. This series of fine vessels—similar to blood vessels—drains fluid away from the tissues and returns it to the bloodstream.

Although there are many different types of lymphoma, the two main ones are Hodgkin's Disease—the type contracted by Shirley McCallum—and non-Hodgkin's Lymphoma. In some cases the former has been linked to an infection known as the Epstein-Barr virus, which, although very common, actually causes relatively few of those infected to go on and develop Hodgkin's Disease. The incidence of non-Hodgkin's Lymphoma is rising, although the cause or causes of this disease are poorly understood at the moment. A small percentage of cases occur in people whose immune systems are not working properly—perhaps after a transplant, or because they have HIV infection.

In both forms of the disease, the first sign is usually swollen glands or lymph nodes, often in the neck. Other symptoms may include persistent fever, severe night sweats, persistent tiredness, unexplained weight loss or generalised itchy skin. In the case of Hodgkin's Disease statistics show the peak ages for contracting the disease are from 15 to 30 years, and a second peak occuring over age 50.

Radiotherapy, chemotherapy and stem cell transplantation—which involves replacing the patient's bone marrow with either his or her own own stem cells or from a donor—are the main forms of treatment for lymphoma. Most patients with Hodgkin's Disease can now be cured, and an increasingly large proportion of patients with non-Hodgkin's Lymphoma go on to beat the disease.

Over the past 20 years, a great deal of valuable research has been carried out by doctors belonging to the Scotland and Newcastle Lymphoma Group (SNLG). The group volunteer their time and their expertise is available to all Scotland's hospitals. Dr Lilian Matheson, consultant clinical oncologist at the Western General Hospital in Edinburgh, and Group Treasurer, said up to £100,000 is needed annually to keep their research programme going.

"We currently have no central funding for our data managers and secretarial staff who are essential for our work," she explained. "All patients in Scottish hospitals can benefit from the expertise of the doctors who volunteer their time to the SNLG. Without the Group, we estimate that thousands of patients would be worse off.

"The Group has made major advances and is now recognised as one of the world's leading lights in the pursuit of a cure for lymphoma. Currently 80 per cent of young adults with Hodgkin's Disease beat the illness, but sadly, Shirley was not one of the lucky ones.

"Despite the aggressiveness of her disease, she bounced back many times and astonished the medical staff with her bravery and positive attitude. I sometimes felt there was little I could contribute to her care but Shirley usually proved me wrong.

"We believe that the story of this remarkable young woman will inspire people in a similar position, and hope it will motivate others to support fund-raising efforts, enabling our vital research to continue. Every donation, however great or small, is greatly appreciated and makes a big difference to our work."

STATISTICS from the University of Edinburgh Medical School's Public Health Sciences department show that Hodgkin's Disease is an important disease in young people in Scotland, especially young men. Between 1986 and 1995, it was the the second most common cancer in males aged between 15 and 34, and was one of the top five cancers in females under age 34. During the same period, there was an average of 75 new cases each year in males and 58 in females. Twenty-one male and 19 female deaths were recorded in this time.

Survival rates at five years have continued to increased substantially since 1968: of those cases registered between 1988 and 1992, 75 per cent of males and nearly 70 per cent of females survived after five years, compared with only around 50 per cent for both sexes three decades ago.

[Information courtesy of Dr Freda Alexander, Public Health Sciences, University of Edinburgh Medical School].

For further information, contact:

- Compassionate Friends Helpline (support and friendship for bereaved parents): 0117 966 5202
- Finbar Nolan, Faith Healer, 12 Trafalgar Terrace, Seapoint, Co. Dublin (00 3531 280 2542).
- Leukaemia Research Fund, 43 Great Ormond Street, London (0171 405 0101).
- Scotland and Newcastle Lymphoma Group (PALS Volunteers), Room 666, University of Edinburgh Medical School, Teviot Place, Edinburgh: Sheila MacLaren (01316504382).
- Our Way—Travel Indurance Specialist (travel insurance for people with medical/physical disadvantages): Foxbury House, Foxbury Road, Bromley, Kent BR1 4DG, United Kingdom. Tel: 0181 313 3353; Fax: 0181 313 3652; e-mail: ourwayins@aol.com

Acknowledgements

Publication of "A Quiet Courage" would not have been possible without help, advice and moral support from:

Carol Bell

Borders General Hospital

Mo and Ian Brown

Walter Elliot

Archie Mackay, Special Projects Editor, Sunday Mail

Macmillan Nurses

Staff at Allied Builders Merchants Ltd.

Public Health Sciences,
University of Edinburgh Medical School

James and Cath Rutherford

Sir Michael and Lady Strang Steel

Western General Hospital, Oncology Department

Gordon Webster

Gwen Fabris

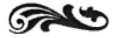

Mary Wormell

Lightning Source UK Ltd.
Milton Keynes UK
UKOW050303080312

188553UK00003B/24/P